PLANNING FOR MEDICAL RESEARCH:

A practical guide to research methods

DEREK LOWE

First Published in Great Britain by
Astraglobe Limited
in 1993

ii

To my wife Sophia,
and to my parents Elsie & Hubert Lowe

Printed in Great Britain by Antony Rowe Ltd, Chippenham, Wiltshire

ISBN 0 9522839 0 5

Published by:
Astraglobe Limited
24 Trinity Place
Congleton
Cheshire CW12 3JB
United Kingdom

Fax: 01260 278396

Astraglobe Limited, Registered in Cardiff, No 2804927
Reg Office: 24 Trinity Place, Congleton, Cheshire CW12 3JB

CONTENTS

PREFACE

I have worked hard to make this novel book useful for the reference shelves of medical researchers. It's novel because it constantly relates to you at the stage when you are putting together a research plan, or protocol. It covers both design and analysis.

You may be a postgraduate student thinking about a research project for your course. Or you might be employed in a medical or para-medical profession and have an idea for research you wish to take further. Or you could be employed in a research capacity and wish to broaden your understanding of research methodology. Or you may be involved in audit work . Whether beginner or experienced dabbler, if you are about to undertake medical research or audit and you are unsure how best to plan it, this book can be of help to you. It will identify most things concerning design and analysis that you need to think about at the planning stage and will help you avoid the most obvious traps.

There have been quite a few textbooks on statistical methods for medical research in the last few years and although I am a statistician the emphasis in this book is on research methodology rather than on methods of statistical analysis. One of the saddest aspects of being a statistician is being unable to rescue a poorly designed study by pulling a magical statistical analysis out of the hat. The true meaning of results often has more to do with non-statistical considerations than with the way data are analysed.

I've tried to avoid bogging you down in detail, of losing sight of the wood because of the trees, which is a common problem with weighty texts. It is very important that you retain the overall vision of what you are trying to do when you read this book. Many things have to come right and together to capture a meaningful answer to a research question.

This is not a textbook, more a practical clarification of issues. Such issues generalise across disciplines, and the book is therefore suitable for both hospital and community based researchers. It is a practical guidebook you can refer to time and time again as you take on new research.

I draw on my experience of many hundreds of consultations and co-operations with health professionals from a variety of disciplines who were engaged in research work. The principles of good study design are common to most health service disciplines and I have attempted to convey these principles in a simple style free of technical, algebraic or statistical jargon. Examples clarify the main principles involved.

The vast majority of examples in the book arise from my involvements in community and hospital research. They have been "doctored" so as to trim your attention to the essential points being made. I see no need for you to be caught up in irrelevant and unnecessary technicalities. I also wish to retain the comprehension and interest of readers from across the disciplines.

As you read from cover to cover, make notes to yourself. These will be questions, comments or future actions. Most open questions should resolve as you progress through the book. Each chapter ends with a reference to further reading.

1. INITIAL THOUGHTS

Introduction

Research means different things to different people. To some it may imply a large scale undertaking lasting many years with a full-time team and back-up resources. For others it might merely be looking a little deeper into something that interests them. For all of us though, research is about finding answers to questions.

A good researcher doesn't try and cut too many corners. Data collection and analysis come relatively late in the day and research of value may well depend on very careful preparation stretching over many months. Write down your plans for research in some detail. Call this the research proposal or protocol and let it reflect current thoughts. Your first protocol will be a short statement of intent, a skeleton outline. Subsequent protocols add on the flesh.

Why Bother with a Research Protocol?

It may seem unnecessarily pedantic to have to describe each step of the research in detail but it is worth it. It is a little like setting out to build yourself a house. However experienced you are in such matters it would be foolhardy to attempt such a project without a very detailed plan of action, a written plan that could be shown to others, particularly for expert comment and approval. Otherwise you could find yourself buried under a pile of rubble.

Those wonderful ideas floating around in your head should be written down since otherwise they will drift away. Gaps and flaws become easier to spot when it is all laid out in black and white. A written protocol allows others to take in your ideas at their leisure and to come up with constructive criticism. Some comments may be unhelpful, but by canvassing a wide spectrum of opinion you will be able to develop a better research strategy. Seek out those with experience in research methods. It is in the planning stages when they can be of most use to you. Get their comments on your protocol. At least promise yourself a visit to your friendliest statistician once you have digested the contents of this book and put together the best written protocol you can

Once your study is underway then your protocol becomes a source of reference allowing for consistency of approach. A protocol protects against fuzziness of memory and changes in personnel. It provides a written representation of what should be going on thereby letting others know exactly what you are doing at the time you are doing it. The detail should be sufficient for researchers elsewhere to be able to replicate your work. Also it provides the base for the writing up and presentation of work at the end of the project, particularly the introduction and method sections.

There should be a clear link running through the whole protocol from the statements of problem and purpose, through the type of study and sampling methods to the variables measured, the mode of analysis and the sample size. The analysis of accurate data using the chosen research design should be clearly seen to satisfactorily address the main purpose of the study.

The keywords in table 1.1 give a flavour and a structure for the rest of this book. Subsequent chapters expand on these aspects of study design. When preparing a study protocol each keyword should be thought about carefully, though some may not necessarily apply to the study you have in mind.

Funding bodies have their own reviewing procedures and applications are often rejected because they give the impression that the study has been poorly thought through. A funding body tries to ensure through expert advice that a research proposal lays out appropriate goals, that the methodology described will be suitable to achieve these goals, and consequently that the results will be scientifically acceptable. A well thought out protocol provides the information needed to complete any grant application with relative ease and confidence.

Submit your protocol to your local ethical committee whose responsibilities particularly concern the misuse of patients,

Table 1.1 KEYWORDS

STATEMENT OF PROBLEM
BACKGROUND & LITERATURE REVIEW
MAIN PURPOSE OF STUDY
TARGET AND STUDY POPULATIONS

TYPE OF STUDY		
	prospective	case-control
	cross-sectional	case-series
	retrospective	clinical trial
	longitudinal	incidence
	experiment	prevalence
	cohort	survey

SAMPLING:		
	simple random sampling	REPRESENTATION
	systematic	RANDOM METHODS
	stratified	BIAS
	cluster	
	convenience	

CONTROL OF VARIABLES: - selection criteria
                         - matching
                         - randomization
                         - stratification
                         - double-blinding

DATA MEASUREMENT & COLLECTION: -how/when/by whom/where

    Which Variables?
    VALIDITY
    RELIABILITY

DATA SUMMARY: : tables/pictures/summary statistics

STATISTICAL INFERENCE: - confidence intervals
                        - significance tests

SAMPLE SIZE: - required precision for statistical inference
                       - statistical power.

OTHER: - ethical aspects (eg informed consent)
                       - PILOT study
                       - staff/timetable/facilities/equipment/
                       supplies/travel/money

        ASK: WHY WHEN HOW WHO WHAT WHERE

healthy volunteers, animals and other resources. Their concern extends to the way your study is designed. A bad study design is bad ethics and a waste of public resources.

Development of problem

The introduction to a protocol can be thought of as an essay weaving together various strands in a logical sequence:

Initial problem or question
Literature review
Theories, explanations, untested Links
Hypotheses
Target & study populations
Purpose of intended research
Speculation as to outcome of research

Initial question(s)

What was the original problem or question? How and why did it occur? Problems can be expressed as questions, as for example in the following General Practice study concerned with the problems of patient non-compliance to a new drug:

What are the demographic characteristics of non-compliant patients for whom I prescribe drug A?

What is the relationship between (occupational) social class and the level of compliance to drug A therapy?

Why do my patients from higher social classes appear to have a poor level of drug A compliance?

Questions beginning with *what is* or *what are* require a descriptive answer. They suggest little or no information on the topic in question is available to the researcher. Questions beginning with *what is the relationship between* suggest perhaps that the topics concerned have been studied before, though possibly not together in the context proposed. Questions beginning with *why* suggest perhaps that previous work has been done with some noteworthy finding being reported. The question is now why such a finding should be so and from an extensive literature review, countless discussions, combined with your own gut feelings, you might be able to come up with some theoretical *because* answer. To test out your theory you may be able to re-express the *why* question into one of the other two types of question, as for example:

> What are the reasons given for non-compliance by patients from each occupational social class?

A clear statement of what the research is about will help to focus your attention on the most appropriate choice of methods for your study. Make sure you are very clear as to the questions you want answering. Write them down in your protocol.

Background and literature review

Get in touch with people who have relevant knowledge you can tap. Besides helping you formulate your ideas they may provide you with suggestions for your literature review. Use the review also as an opportunity to assess appropriate research methods.

The relevance of any pertinent findings, published or unpublished, should be written into your protocol. Leave out the irrelevant material. Other people will read your protocol so spare them the agony. The same goes for grant applications. Few will be impressed by a demonstration of depth and breadth of reading. So be comprehensive in your reading but relevant and concise in summary for others.

Picture the drunk who leans on the street lamp for support rather than for illumination. It almost goes without saying that this part of the protocol should be a fair balance of work already done. Yet this has to be said since it is all too easy to get carried away through strong conviction. How you view the work of others may well vary according to your awareness of research and statistical methods. It could be that after reading this book you will weigh the balance of evidence somewhat differently.

Consult your nearest librarian for help and guidance in your search for material. A librarian can suggest pathways you may never think of for yourself. Various computer library search systems exist. There is a wealth of routine statistical information available at local, regional, national and international level. There are estimates of population size, birth and death rates, notifiable diseases rates, hospital inpatient statistics, ad-hoc morbidity surveys in general practice and so forth.

Have regard to the kind of people who will be reading your protocol and word your document accordingly. When putting together an application for money avoid specialist jargon as much as possible. The more people that can understand you the better. This also applies to saying why it is important for you to do the research. What seems like stating the obvious to you may not appear as such to someone else unless you clearly spell it out.

Making sense of it all

Weave together all the background material to form the introduction and then, if possible, supply some underlying theory or explanation to link together the various strands you have accumulated.

Development of theories helps to identify ambiguous and untested strands. These are ripe for study and lead to the formation of specific study hypotheses. Write down the hypotheses you will investigate.

A hypothesis is little more than an educated guess about the nature of the relationship between two or more variables. For example:

> Individuals from lower occupational social classes are less likely to use primary health care services than those from higher social classes

The two variables involved in this hypothesis are occupational social class and the use of primary health care services. These variables will have to be measured for the hypothesis to be investigated and there may be more than one view as to how each should be measured. Well-constructed hypotheses will involve variables that have the potential for being accurately measured. Hypotheses are essentially of three kinds:

1) there is no relationship between variables
2) the direction of a relationship is known
3) a relationship is suspected but the direction is unknown.

Some studies aim to describe the whole group surveyed - for example a series of questions asking patients about their level of satisfaction with the services offered by a family planning clinic. There might be speculation about whether the satisfaction level will be high or low but unless two or more variables are involved (eg age and satisfaction level) then these speculations shouldn't be referred to as hypotheses.

Examples of Hypotheses:

1) There is no association between age and satisfaction level

2) Younger clients are less satisfied with the service provided than older clients.

3) There is an association between age and satisfaction level.

Defining relevant populations

The *target* population comprises those subjects you are really interested in generalising the results of analysis to. A sample is usually chosen from the *study* population which sometimes forms only part of the target population. For example the target population might be all people under the age of 30 years who have Down's Syndrome. The study group might comprise all those people under the age of 30 years who have Down's Syndrome and who live in an institutional environment within one health district. The difference between the two types of population lie in the compromises being made between trying to be fully representative on the one hand and realistic with available resources on the other.

Give as much detail as possible as to who qualifies to be in your target and study populations. Who would you wish to exclude? Define your exclusion rules carefully and then you will find it easier to remain consistent in your selection of a sample. You will also know more clearly the boundaries when you eventually find yourself in the happy position of being able to interpret your study results.

> The purpose is to test the hypothesis that children referred to Speech Therapy Services under the age of three and a half years respond equally well to a home based therapy programme as to the more traditional clinic based programme

The above statement of purpose loosely defines a target population. Now suppose various initial (or baseline) assessments are carried out and that the results of these are to be used to exclude the following groups of children from further participation in the research:

> Exclude Children with:
>
> a. A severe motor disorder requiring special educational placement
>
> b. A profound hearing loss requiring special educational placement.
>
> c. Mental retardation requiring special educational placement.
>
> d. Severe disorder of the use of language, eg autism, requiring special educational placement.

The target population has thus been refined though its boundaries still lack precision since the criteria for severe, profound and so on require further definition.

Imagine now that a study population that is made up of children satisfying all the above selection criteria and who live in one locality and who are referred to one of two speech therapists.

The study sample comes from this local study population and it is to the study population that any conclusions drawn from the sample can most legitimately be applied. Inference from study to target population becomes more speculative.

The inferential process from sample to study population is complicated if the study population includes people who refuse to take part in the study, and people who withdraw (or drop out) after the research begins. Those intended for but lost to study may be quite unlike those that remain and this could affect the conclusions drawn from the study as a whole. Consider now this next example:-

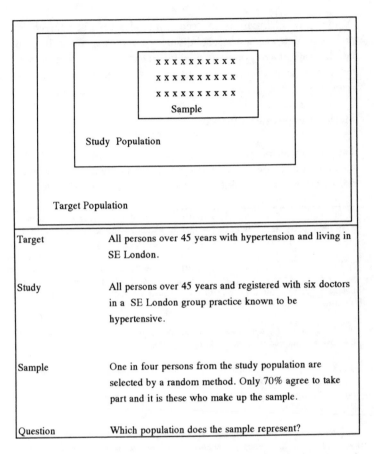

Target	All persons over 45 years with hypertension and living in SE London.
Study	All persons over 45 years and registered with six doctors in a SE London group practice known to be hypertensive.
Sample	One in four persons from the study population are selected by a random method. Only 70% agree to take part and it is these who make up the sample.
Question	Which population does the sample represent?

In the early stages of protocol development a rough outline of the study population is all that is needed. You can become more precise as more detailed plans are made.

Practical considerations in the choice of study population include the minimising of travel by researchers, the accessibility, and the degree of co-operation to be expected from subjects. Researchers often commit themselves too early to small convenient populations with the justification of homogeneity (or purity).

A good rule of thumb is to keep as broad a base of subjects as possible. You can always subdivide your data analysis if need be. If your study population is far removed from your target population then you will have difficulty convincing others of the relevance of your research.

Stating the purpose of study

The statement of purpose represents the culmination of the introduction. In one or two sentences it says what you intend to do, where you intend to do it, and with whom. For example:

1) The purpose of the study is to report the prevalence of dental caries in a population of 6 year old children resident in, and attending schools in, SE inner London.

2) The purpose of the study is to investigate the hypothesis that patients with high initial resistance to dietary therapy are less likely to comply with the dietary program offered by nutritionists at hospital Z than patients with low initial response.

3) The purpose of the study is to establish the incidence of deep vein thrombosis in burned patients attending the burns unit at hospital X.

4) The study will measure smoking cessation in chronic heavy smokers employed by health authority X. In a randomized experiment the purpose of the study is to investigate the hypothesis that acupuncture helps cessation both in the shorter and longer term.

5) The purpose of the randomized experiment in hospital Z is to investigate the hypothesis that the giving of epidural analgesia to mothers in labour has beneficial effects for the small for dates foetus.

6) The purpose of the audit is to report the number of medical and surgical admissions that require High Dependency Unit (HDU) care at S. Hospital (which doesn't have an HDU Unit) for each day of a four week period in October and to use this information to review the need for a HDU unit.

Background reading and discussions will have clarified the research problem and hopefully given a feel for appropriate research methods. The statement of purpose points out the direction of the study. You are now ready to map out the plan of action and to flesh out the details.

Speculating about the outcome of the research

The importance of having research questions you set out to answer might at first read seem obvious but it cannot be emphasised enough. There is a great temptation to over-analyse data, i.e. to torture it. Tortured data may well confess something in some obscure subgroup of subjects but how honest would such a finding be? The results of such torture may be worth reporting but should be separated and relegated in importance from those results which directly relate to questions posed at the beginning of the study and before any data were collected. Consider the following:

> You, me, him & her are playing whist and I have just shuffled the pack. I deal 13 cards to each of us. You pick up your cards and discover you have 11 hearts and hearts are trumps.
>
> Afterwards we all agreed that your remarkable hand of cards could only have occurred by chance since we had already played several unspectacular hands and the cards had been well shuffled.
>
> It would however have been a far more remarkable turn of events if you had predicted such a good hand before I had dealt the cards out.

You should only expect to discover those things you have set out to discover. State your expectations in your protocol.

Such prior speculation as to future outcome is the basis on which good research is rooted. The ability to speculate derives from a thorough background and literature review, a full development of the problem, and a refinement of often rather vague initial questions into specific statements of purpose. This process is a healthy foundation for identifying the research problems that exist.

It could be said that speculation on the outcome of a study might actually influence or bias the workings of the study and hence its results. With a poorly designed study this could be true. The design you finally adopt should be as free as possible from bias. In approach it should be seen to adopt the stance of neutrality and objectivity. All researchers probably do have biased views and know what sort of results they would like to see and thus great care has to be taken to prevent the research swaying in that direction.

Further reading (See Chapter 9 for full list of references):

Ref 5 (chpt 3)
Ref 6 (p22-25)
Ref 24

2. TYPES OF STUDY

Study the language of this chapter carefully and adopt its terms for your subsequent use. Write them into your protocol to describe your choice of design. Speak them when you discuss your methodology with others. As you read this chapter you must constantly try to relate the issues to your own planning. In particular pay attention to potential problems with each type of design. As you perceive a problem for your own research think about how you might resolve it. In this and later chapters you will learn how to avoid many difficulties. Some designs will be unsuited for your study but please read the whole chapter as this will sharpen your awareness in general.

Some researchers set out to describe, some attempt to explain, whilst others experiment. The final choice of design will depend on the current level of knowledge, on the resources available, on whether the purpose of the study is primarily to observe or to intervene and on the likely access to and co-operation from relevant populations. A number of terms, often overlapping, are commonly used to describe study design, and Figure 2.1 illustrates these.

Cross-sectional and Longitudinal studies

In a cross-sectional study measurements on a subject are made more or less at one point in time. In a longitudinal study measurements on a subject are made over a period of time. The difference between the two can be likened to the difference between taking a snapshot (cross-sectional) and making a video (longitudinal).

Imagine a study to find out the level of hypertension in a population of patients aged 45 years and over and who are registered with one general practice in SE London.

For practical reasons it would be difficult for every patient to be seen at one single point in time, eg on the morning of May 24th. If a patient's blood pressure is found to be high then that person would most likely be seen again (and then possibly again) for confirmation of hypertensive status.

The study might thus take several months to complete. Although the data would be collected on more than one occasion (repeat visits) or at different times for different people, the study is cross-sectional. The intention is to make some statement about the current hypertensive status (current snapshot) of each person and all the data collected for each person is used to produce such an assessment.

If each of the subjects were to be seen again 5 years later and their hypertensive status re-assessed the interest of the study would focus on changes over time. Such a study would be longitudinal.

Classifying a study as either cross-sectional or longitudinal doesn't directly depend on the time period covered by the measurements. Elapsed calendar time can be regarded as either a means to an end (to establish a current status) or as an object of main interest.

If you undertake cross-sectional work then be concerned about the validity of data you will collect, the adequacy of your method of sampling from a population, and issues of bias & representativeness. Bias could come from an unrepresentative sample, a badly worded questionnaire, unstandardised interviewers, examiners or observers and through non-response. Longitudinal studies have the added administrative burden of following up subjects. Other biases that can creep up on you are those due to subject migration and the withdrawal of subject co-operation.

Figure 2.1 Types of Study

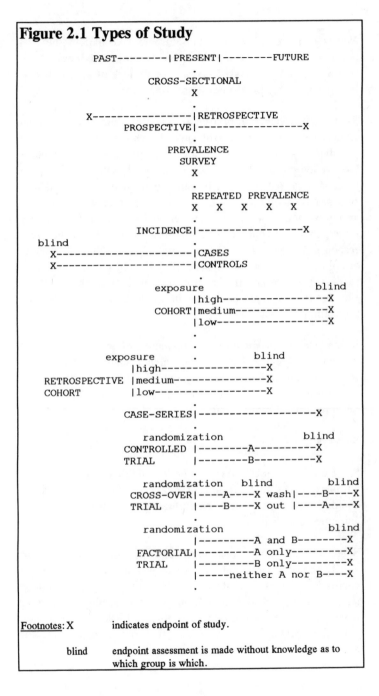

```
                PAST--------|PRESENT|--------FUTURE
                                .
                        CROSS-SECTIONAL
                              X
                                .
            X----------------|RETROSPECTIVE
                PROSPECTIVE|----------------X
                                .
                         PREVALENCE
                           SURVEY
                              X
                                .
                        REPEATED  PREVALENCE
                        X    X    X    X    X
                                .
                    INCIDENCE|----------------X
        blind                   .
          X----------------------|CASES
          X----------------------|CONTROLS
                                .
                    exposure                 blind
                        |high----------------X
                 COHORT|medium--------------X
                        |low-----------------X
                                .
                                .
                exposure        .       blind
                        |high----------------X
        RETROSPECTIVE  |medium--------------X
        COHORT         |low-----------------X
                                .
                    CASE-SERIES|------------------X
                    randomization            blind
                    CONTROLLED |--------A----------X
                    TRIAL      |--------B----------X
                                .
                    randomization    blind        blind
                    CROSS-OVER|----A----X wash|----B----X
                    TRIAL     |----B----X out |----A----X
                                .
                    randomization            blind
                            |---------A and B-------X
                    FACTORIAL|---------A only--------X
                    TRIAL    |---------B only--------X
                            |-----neither A nor B----X
                                .
```

<u>Footnotes:</u> X   indicates endpoint of study.

blind   endpoint assessment is made without knowledge as to which group is which.

Non-responders are those who refuse to take part in the first place or are those who later drop out (or withdraw). Non-response may be expressed verbally or by lack of action such as in refusing to complete a questionnaire.

Representativeness can best be achieved by sampling at random from a comprehensive list of subjects who make up the target population, so long as there is a good response and the sample is large enough. Random sampling coupled with a very poor response rate (eg of 50%) is unlikely to give a sample that is representative of the population from which it was drawn. A sample with only a few subjects selected at random from a very large population could also be unrepresentative, even with 100% response, because of the chance variations possible with random sampling. For example suppose 10 UK subjects are chosen at random from census information and all live in the South of England - how representative will their views be of the UK population as a whole?

In many research situations a population of interest cannot be individually identified and a convenience sample from a more accessible population is the only option. In such circumstances the nature of any selection biases will form a crucial part in the interpretation of sample data.

Surveys

Some cross-sectional surveys relate to a single population, eg an attitudes survey of convalescent mothers. Other surveys make comparisons, such as between cultural groups in feeding habits and nutritional beliefs.

Some surveys establish community age-sex norm values, that are ascribed to the general public and which in turn could be used as comparison or control data in future surveys. Thus various characteristics (eg alcohol consumption) of patients suffering from a certain disease might be compared to those of a sample from the general public, with due allowance perhaps made for age and sex.

Surveys often involve interviews and self-completing (sometimes postal) questionnaires but can also involve the scrutiny of existing record systems (eg a survey of patient notes looking for the presence of blood pressure recordings). A big problem with existing record systems is that the variable of interest is unlikely to have been recorded with the purpose of the current research in mind. Always question the accuracy of any data collected for purposes other than your own.

Why does one person respond to a questionnaire survey and another refuse? There are many possible reasons including:

1) Perceived importance of the topic being considered.
2) Subject's age and sex.
3) Subject's social circumstances.
4) Subject's level of education.
5) Subject's health.
6) The style & content of a covering explanatory letter.
7) Confidentiality guarantees.
8) The inclusion of a pre-paid reply.
9) Whether a local or outside organisation is doing the research.
10) The length and complexity of a questionnaire.

Think hard about your study, whatever kind it might be, as to whether any of the above might influence the availability of the data you want to collect.

Whatever your study design you should regard a response rate of under 90% as unsatisfactory. Those who respond will be different in certain respects to those who refuse. You won't know how they might differ unless you make repeated efforts to persuade a higher proportion to respond. The comparison of early with late respondents in analysis may help throw some light on the nature of any bias resulting from non-response. A 90% response is often difficult to achieve and the last 15% can be harder to get than the first 75%.

Experimental and Observational Studies

An experimental study involves an evaluation of some deliberate intervention, this intervention (eg drug, surgery) having been introduced into the study specifically to address the purpose of the study.

An observational study is one in which naturally occurring events are measured. These events may include interventions such as the giving of drugs but there is an important distinction to be made since such interventions are out of the direct control of the researcher.

An example of an experiment is one in which patients with lung function difficulties are randomly allocated either to receive a course of drug therapy or to receive no drug therapy, with all patients being followed-up for 5 years. The hypothesis is that the drug will reduce the decline in lung function (as measured by FEV_1) to half that expected without drug therapy. The random allocation of patients to either receive drug therapy or to receive no drug therapy is a deliberate act of intervention specifically to further the purpose of the study.

An example of an observational study is one that describes the relationship between smoking status and the lung function profile of subjects drawn from a general practice population and who are observed longitudinally over time. Some patients may receive medication during their period of observation but this would be entirely at the discretion of the medical professionals concerned and not in any way influenced or manipulated by the researcher.

Prospective and Retrospective Studies

A prospective study is a longitudinal study that begins at the present time and moves forward into future time. A retrospective study considers the past and can be longitudinal.

An example of a longitudinal retrospective study is one that uses a previously defined comprehensive population, for example the population of all graduating dentists for 1961. A sample from the list is traced to the present day and an examination of hearing status carried out. A group of graduating doctors also for 1961 provides a useful control group in a study to assess the extent of hearing loss in dentists. The basis for sample selection belongs in the past but the emphasis is on change over time.

A retrospectively chosen cohort aims to steal a march on time though in this study of hearing loss in dentists the exposure to noise, particularly drills, would most likely have to be obtained retrospectively from the cohort by questions asked at the present time. A study like this is susceptible to biases of memory loss and exaggeration and of record systems designed for some other purpose.

In a prospective study more control is possible over the collection of data and a more valid answer is likely though the study would clearly take longer to do. A quick retrospective study can provide ammunition for arguing the case for a prospective study.

Cohort, Case series, and Case-Control Studies

Cohort

In a cohort study subjects are followed in time and are initially selected because of some known exposure, or degree of exposure, to some factor of interest. The follow-up of all subjects allows for a comparison between exposure groups in the occurrence of defined endpoints. The provision of objective evidence of exposure is essential. A cohort study is longitudinal and either prospective or retrospective (as in a cohort of dentists graduating in 1961). Many cohort studies use cohorts of subjects which are easily obtainable, such as various professions and workforces for which a register, record system or pay-roll system is kept. Maternity records are another source from which a cohort of babies or of mothers can be obtained. Hospital patient information systems could be used to give a cohort of patients admitted to hospital.

The analysis of cohort study data concentrates on the measurement of risk. The association between the study endpoint and its suspected determinants or causal agents is measured as risk. Thus we talk of risk factors. Make sure you measure all known key prognostic variables. The chance you take with any observational study when attempting to establish causality is that alternative explanations are always possible. For example:

Breast Cancer has various known risk factors. Age is one of these, as is country lived in, and age at menarche & menopause. Socio-economic status is another and so is family history. The association of breast cancer with socio-economic status may well suggest that affluent living, perhaps diet, is a main cause of breast cancer. Associations to do with reproduction suggest hormonal influences, whilst associations with family history suggest some genetic component.

A risk factor could be a causal agent but more likely, as above, it reflects some underlying agent which itself is correlated (associated) with both the risk factor and the endpoint of interest.

The measurement of risk invites comparison. Do smokers carry a higher risk of developing emphysema than non-smokers, and what about ex-smokers? The risk in one subgroup is expressed relative to the risk in another subgroup, and the resultant measure is known as relative risk.

A single cohort may inherently possess the comparison groups of interest, as for example a birth cohort with comparison groups defining maternal smoking habits during pregnancy (eg none/day, 1-9 cigs/day, 10+ cigs/day). Valid exposure data is of course vital so that the cohort of children can be subgrouped according to the degree of exposure. A dose-response analysis by (developmental) outcome of the child is then possible.

When a cohort is entirely defined by its exposure to a possible causal agent then some external control is sought. It is sometimes difficult to identify the most appropriate control group and whatever selection criteria are finally employed these will be crucial in the final interpretation of results:

Imagine a study cohort comprising all those people on a national register and who are known at the present time to have a particular disease. The study hypothesis is that people with this disease have a different pattern of mortality, especially an increase in deaths from certain cancers because of their long-term treatment with a certain kind of drug. The cohort mortality experience would thus be monitored over the period of observation for the study.

There may be patients on a similar but different disease register who are unlikely to be exposed to the drug in question. These at least would provide some control for being known on a disease register.

The mortality experience of the disease cohort(s) can also be compared with the expected mortality for the general population over the same calendar time period. The expected mortality experience for a cohort can be computed by reference to published national mortality data subdivided by age, sex, and calendar year.

In the UK you can get details about a person's death from the NHS Central Register in Southport. If the Central Register is given certain details about a person, such as their name, last known address, name of GP and NHS number (if known) then that person can be tagged on the register and you will subsequently be informed of death, cancer notification and emigration during the follow-up period of study. Many patients apparently lost to follow-up in a longitudinal study can thus be traced in this way and then accounted for in the results of the research.

Post-marketing surveillance is one kind of cohort study in which 'exposed' persons receiving an established drug are monitored for serious adverse effects.

Case-Series

A *case* usually refers to a patient suffering from some specified disease or condition, and a prospective case-series is a cohort of patients. Take care to verify any diagnosis.

An example of a prospective case-series study is a consecutive series of patients admitted to a neurosurgical unit and diagnosed as having had a subarachnoid haemorrhage. Patients are observed through time with the research focusing on the relationship between early time trends in cerebral blood flow and the outcome of the patient 3 months after the haemorrhage.

An example of a retrospective case-series study is a series of patients diagnosed with subarachnoid haemorrhage whose next of kin, close relatives and friends are asked about potential risk factors leading up to the haemorrhage. In this case series a search is made for factors common to most or all of the series. The problem however is the lack of comparison. There is a need here for a control series, and thus a case-control study. Perhaps a control subject of the same age and sex and living in the same street or neighbourhood as a case patient could be sought and surveyed in exactly the same way.

A cross-sectional case-series study could take the form of a survey of subarachnoid haemorrhage survivors interviewed after 3 months survival about their fears of another haemorrhage.

Case-Control

Emphasis is usually placed on past events and because of this the case-control study is referred to as being retrospective. For example:

> A Case-Control study is to be set up to describe the habits and activities of children in relation to the laboratory isolation of cryptosporidia. Cases are those children for whom cryptosporidia is isolated from faecal specimens. One control group comprises children with diarrhoea due to an organism other than cryptosporidia. A second control group comprises children who are well. Parents of case and control children are asked about current and previous behavioural habits of their children. The case and control groups can then be compared in respect of answers received.

The decision to classify a subject as a case or as a control should be backed up by as much verifying information as possible, otherwise the results can get watered down through misclassification. The same attention should be given to providing accurate information about the potential risk factors under study.

Case-control studies allow a relatively quick, cheap and dirty look at suspected risk factors. Relevant information can often be found in existing record systems or can be obtained from survey questionnaires, interviews and clinical examinations. Retrospective data carry problems of memory recall, incompleteness and unstandardised observations and one should be extremely wary of such data.

Cases are often patients admitted to hospital with a certain disease. It is best to include only those newly diagnosed cases, as existing cases may be different in that they still have the disease but have neither been cured of it nor died from it. Also, a patient with a longer-standing illness will have had more time to dwell on the possible causes, is likely to have a more extensive knowledge of the disease and a more immediate recall of past events thought relevant. A new case has less time for inner reflection, and certain past happenings, unless they are probed for carefully, will go undetected.

Controls are often patients in hospital for some unrelated condition, assessed over the same time period of study as the cases. Some case-control studies use more than one control group, for example one hospital control sample and one community sample, and this approach is to be encouraged.

	Travelled abroad in last year:
Hospital Cases	45%
Hospital Controls	40%
Community Controls	20%

The type of control chosen is critical in the interpretation of results, and one should always ask whether hospitalisation in itself for patients has a disturbing (or confounding) influence on the case-control comparisons to be made.

An all too easy option seems to be the recruitment of healthy volunteers to act as *normal* controls. Always question the representativeness of hospital volunteer samples, in particular members of staff. In general the more selective the groups chosen, cases or controls, the less secure any generalisations are likely to be. Community controls, however, are harder to identify and suitable subjects are more likely to refuse to participate. In using invasive techniques as part of your research you may have few options available, but nevertheless the above comments still apply.

The same diagnostic procedure should be applied to all study subjects with the purpose of ensuring that those in the control group are indeed free of the condition being studied. This is important in diseases such as cancer for which disease can occur in asymptomatic form thus avoiding detection unless intentionally sought.

It is very important that case and control data be collected over the same study period. Otherwise temporal changes (such as staff changes and finer tuning of research approach) could account for part or all of those results you find so interesting. So avoid, for example, assessing all your cases before assessing your controls. Mix them up over the study period.

A desirable design feature of any comparative study is that of *blindness*. Those involved in making assessments in a case-control study should ideally be unaware of the status (case or control) of each subject studied:

> Imagine a study to investigate the risk factors of subarachnoid haemorrhage. If you know you are talking to a patient who has had a subarachnoid haemorrhage (case) or to someone from the community neighbourhood close to the case (control) then this knowledge might subconsciously cloud your probing for relevant information, particularly if you know the sort of results you would like to see from your research. It would be better to employ someone who knows nothing about the clinical features of these subjects to probe into their backgrounds to look for possible risk factors. You would have to find some way of preventing subjects from revealing their clinical state to the interviewer, or of recruiting an interviewer from an independent organisation who is unaware of the true purpose of the study.

In some studies blindness will be difficult to achieve. The burden falls on you the researcher to achieve blindness wherever possible and failing this to be able to convince others that blindness is unachievable or undesirable. Lack of blindness is a serious design issue especially when it is avoidable.

Matching techniques can sometimes be used to select a control group with similar matching characteristics:

> For each mother of a baby born with a certain abnormality (cases) the next and previous mothers on the maternity register of the same age with non-affected babies are chosen as controls.

Several controls are preferable to a single control. The matching process in general can be quite time consuming and as the number of matching variables increases so does the number of subjects you need to consider for being a control. More than 4 matching variables is hardly ever practicable. If your case is a mother of 27, from occupational social class 1, living in Congleton CW12 postcode area, and with a family history of hypertension then you will use up a lot of time and energy trying to find another mother from Congleton CW12 of similar age, class and without a family history of hypertension. Likewise for your other cases.

Avoid matching for variables that are under investigation in the research. Thus in the above example if socio-economic risk factors are of interest you wouldn't think of matching on factors such as occupation and income, otherwise you would find little difference between the two groups. Alternatively if diet was of interest as a risk factor you might try to match mothers by socio-economic factors so as to control for any association between socio-economic status and diet. Over-matching could lead to an under-estimation of relative risk.

Matched or *paired* statistical analyses are possible to most efficiently squeeze out a resulting message.

Cohort or case-control ?

The distinction between Cohort and Case-Control studies is helped by considering where the choice of subjects (the sampling) fits into the process of underlying time. Sampling on the basis of an outcome or endpoint (eg disease occurrence, death) will give you a case-control study. Sampling on the basis of some entry point or input (eg birth, drug administration) will allow a longitudinal cohort study in which outcome or endpoint data can be subsequently collected.

Case-control studies in general suffer from the potential criticism that any differences, or any similarities, between case and control groups in the results might in part or whole be due to the way in which the groups, the control group in particular, were chosen.

A prospective cohort study tends to be much more expensive and time consuming than either a retrospective cohort or a case-control study. A prospective study should give a more reliable answer, though it does run the risk that the hypothesis generated might be out of date by the time the study finishes. There is also the challenge of minimising the loss to follow-up. Some prospective studies take decades to report. Others take hardly any time at all, the time being influenced by:

1) Length of intended follow-up.
2) Relative frequency of exposure subgroups (and the time needed to recruit enough subjects in the smallest subgroup).
3) Occurrence (or incidence) of disease or other endpoint of interest.

Cohort studies often require a large number of subjects especially if the condition under investigation is quite rare, and the case-control approach is better suited to very rare diseases. Extremely rare diseases are best described individually as *case-reports*.

You can use a case-control study to first consider a wide range of variables as potential risk factors. In this way the range of variables might be narrowed. This can lead to specific hypotheses being generated for investigation in a prospective cohort study. A prospective study has the advantage of being able to study several different outcomes at once, eg a birth cohort having developmental checks and tests at various times up to and including the first school examination. A number of different risk factors can also be studied in combination so long as they can be identified as subgroups within the cohort.

The sequence of events in a case-control approach is sometimes unclear, as in these three examples:

---

1) A case-control study is to be set-up to look for possible reasons for hearing loss in dentists. A sample of dentists are to be measured to determine hearing status. The cases are those dentists identified by the survey as having hearing loss and these are subdivided into two subgroups: one group with severe hearing loss, the other with moderate or minimal loss. The control group comprises those without loss (allowing for age). Cases and controls are asked about their lifetime experience to noise, particularly the use of drills. This approach allows for a trend in the results to be looked for. Any risk factor is expected to show up most strongly in those with substantial hearing loss and least so in those who have no hearing loss.

However, there still remains the possibility that those with greatest hearing difficulties obtained through dentistry have left the profession altogether, and hence would not appear in a study of this kind.

2) People with respiratory disease (cases) were found to have spent more time in less physically demanding occupations than controls without respiratory disease. Is it more reasonable to suggest that lack of exercise predisposes to respiratory problems, or rather that people with respiratory problems choose to take less demanding jobs, or is it a bit of both?

3) Mothers interviewed after an adverse pregnancy may be more likely to recall events which they perceive could have been associated with such an outcome than mothers whose children were born normally.

A cohort study stands a better chance of distinguishing causes from risk factors.

Incidence and Prevalence studies

The prevalence of a disease is the number of subjects with that disease (ie cases) at a given point in time. The prevalence rate is calculated by dividing the number of cases by the number of subjects at risk of having that disease. A prevalence study is cross-sectional and is useful in the planning of workload and services. If the prevalence rate of a disease was known to vary by age and sex then a projection ahead in time for likely changes in the population structure would allow an estimation of future disease morbidity and workload.

Suppose that a group of General Practitioners wish to discover the prevalence of hypertension in their patients aged 45-64 years. All such patients registered within their group practice are considered to be at risk of having hypertension and they thus comprise the study population. Each patient is identified and a random sample of 200 patients is chosen from the list. Suppose these all agree to take part and that after all the appropriate measurements have been made a total of 60 patients were hypertensive, however so defined. The best estimate of the prevalence rate for the practice 45-64 year olds is thus 60 over 200, that is 30%.

The incidence of a disease is the number of new cases that occur during some defined time period. The incidence risk is calculated by dividing the number of new cases occurring during the time period by the number of subjects at risk of developing the disease during that time. An incidence study is longitudinal and is useful for investigating cause of disease by allowing an estimation of the risk of developing the disease within subgroups of comparative interest.

Consider a study to describe the relationship between patient lifestyle and the development of hypertension. Each patient identified in a cross-sectional prevalence study as being free from hypertension would be monitored at one-yearly intervals so as to allow the calculation of one-year, two-year and subsequent yearly risks of developing hypertension. Initial data regarding lifestyle (such as diet, exercise, leisure, smoking, drinking) taken together with a yearly update of change would allow a comparison of risks of developing hypertension between subgroups of interest.

Note that those initially identified as having hypertension are no longer at risk of developing hypertension and would be excluded from the denominator of the incidence rate calculations. These patients could be monitored longitudinally as a separate group.

Diseases with low incidence can, if they are slow to resolve, have high prevalence at any one time. Prevalence, or amount, thus results from:

1) Occurrence of new cases (incidence)
2) Duration from onset to end of the disease process (resolution)

Thus the prevalence of the common cold results from the incidence of the common cold and the rate of resolution. A bathtub definition is such that the amount of water in the bath represents prevalence, the water flowing into the bath represents incidence, whilst two plug holes at the bottom of the bath represent recovery and death.

The common cold serves as a useful example to distinguish between point and period prevalence. Point prevalence is the usual understanding of prevalence implying the prevalence at one moment or point in time.

Of 50 students 5 have a cold, giving a point prevalence of 10%. Twenty either now have a cold or have had a cold within the last two months, giving a two-month prevalence rate of 40%.

This two month period prevalence for the students is higher than the point prevalence estimate. Those developing more than one cold during the period would only count once towards the numerator in the calculation of prevalence.

In diseases with very short duration a period prevalence is of greater potential use for future resources planning. In diseases of very long duration and low incidence point and period prevalence estimates will not differ all that much.

Note that prevalence and incidence can relate to any event other than disease, such as for example the level of opinion (prevalence), or the rate of change of opinion (incidence) in those who previously held a particular opinion.

In a prospective study the risk in exposed and unexposed groups is measured by the incidence rate. The relative risk of a particular outcome in one subgroup relative to another is thus measured by the ratio of incidence rates. Thus, consider the following conclusion from a clinical trial:

> If the incidence of deep joint sepsis within 1 years after being 'exposed' to a new operation procedure is 1% and the risk from being exposed to the old standard procedure is 2% then the relative risk of the new to old procedures is 0.5. That is, there is a halving of risk of deep joint sepsis through the use of the new procedure.

Another statement of risk is the attributable risk. The risk attributable to exposure is measured by the arithmetic difference between the incidence rates for the exposed and unexposed groups. In the above example:

> The risk attributable to the old procedure is 2%-1%=1%. Thus by adopting the new procedure in place of the old then 1% of all patients so managed will avoid deep joint sepsis within one year of operation.

In a case-control study incidence cannot be directly calculated because the study isn't longitudinal. A simple way to estimate the relative risk in situations when the incidence can be assumed to be low is by computing what is called an odds ratio (see chapter 6).

Repeated Prevalence trend study

A population is repeatedly sampled at different times with each sample giving an estimate of prevalence. The trend in these estimates is of considerable interest.

The intention in a repeated prevalence study isn't to follow the same people through time. The people in the samples at each time point will largely be different, though there might be some overlap. Since each sample is chosen to be representative of some defined population some subjects may by chance have been included on more than one occasion, and this is acceptable.

> A study to describe experiences and opinions of services provided by the Health Authority might be repeated on an annual basis. Each year a sample of service users is chosen from computer files and sent a questionnaire. The population is large in number and each annual sample comprises but a small but hopefully representative fraction of the whole. The interest after the first prevalence study would be in the trends emerging over time.

Populations change over time as people get older, migrate, die or are born. In repeated trend studies alternative explanations of an interesting trend are always possible because of other temporal changes that may have taken place over the time span of the trend. These may alter the composition, experiences, or exposures of one population relative to another.

Experiments

An experiment is when a researcher deliberately intervenes. If human patients are involved the experiment is known as a clinical trial. A true experiment features the random allocation of subjects to one or more intervention groups. In this way roughly the same distribution of age, sex, or of any other variable can be achieved in each group. Thus control (or allowance) for potentially disturbing influences on outcome is possible by ensuring each of the intervention groups is influenced to a similar extent.

Deliberate intervention by researchers raises special ethical issues. There are situations in which manipulation by randomization are unrealistic or unethical, eg the randomization of babies with phenylketenuria to either a low or high protein diet to investigate the hypothesis that a long term high protein diet impairs intellect. An alternative form of study to investigate this hypothesis is a prospective cohort study. Natural variability in compliance to a low protein diet would allow subgroups for comparison to develop over time. One would have to be wary though of possible confounding social variables associated both with compliance and measures of intelligence.

Single intervention group

Suppose a case series of patients presenting with some complaint are given a new form of treatment and are then later assessed as to their condition. If the intention is to evaluate this new treatment then it is difficult to do so without some comparison group of similar patients who don't receive this form of therapy.

Suppose you are to study the effectiveness of a new management procedure at your local hospital in preventing post operative deep vein thrombosis (DVT). Suppose you did a single intervention study and that when you analysed the data 12 % of patients developed DVT. Furthermore suppose that other studies elsewhere reported DVT rates as low as 0 % and as high as 32% for alternative procedures. (Such a variety of results is by no means uncommon even for the same intervention!) By taking a large enough sample you can give a reasonably accurate estimate of the DVT rate in your own hospital and at the end of the day your study might well have achieved an acceptable incidence of DVT.

However you (and other people) would have great difficulty in relating your results to alternative procedures and other hospital situations. There will always be the criticism that an internal comparison group is missing, a comparison group which could give a higher or lower DVT rate for an alternative procedure. Hence doubt will surround any claims made for the effectiveness of the procedure relative to any other procedure. The results might at best serve to generate interest for a controlled, randomized, clinical trial somewhere else.

Data from other recent studies do provide some comparison for results of a single group intervention study but are limited in value. Distant historical data are even worse. So many confounding factors may creep into and distort the comparisons made, many of which can escape comprehension. Systematic errors between different hospitals, centres or research institutions could be very large indeed. Historical data from within the same centre also pose similar kinds of problems for interpretation. Changes in patient case-mix, in selection criteria, in staff and technology, in consistency of approach to measurement and to management are all examples of confounding factors.

Any attempt to evaluate the effect of a particular cure for the common cold in a single group study is confounded (or confused) by the natural resolution of the cold over time. A treatment-free or better still a placebo group of subjects followed in parallel to the treatment group, concurrently in time, provides the model for adequate comparison. By *placebo* is meant a dummy or camouflaged treatment dressed up to look like the real thing. In appearance, taste, touch, smell, and so forth placebo and real treatments should be indistinguishable. This makes the treatments *blind* to the person receiving them and is important particularly if the evaluation of effectiveness rests upon statements from the subject such as feelings about pain, relief of symptoms or side effects.

Ideally a study should be *double-blind* in that neither patient nor research observer is aware of the nature of the intervention for that patient. Professional judgements of a patient's progress may be clouded unconsciously by the knowledge of what the treatment is. Unintentional bias might show in the classification of marginal cases towards the outcomes that support the direction hoped for or expected in the results. Sometimes the very nature of the intervention implies that double-blindness cannot be achieved. A randomized study comparison of daycase and inpatient cataract surgeries cannot be made double-blind since the nature of intervention is clearly known by the patient. It is possible however that any follow-up visual acuity assessments could be made by an independent assessor unaware of which kind of surgery had occurred.

Two or more comparison groups, and the Randomization process

The aim of a randomized experiment is to achieve a comparison of two or more intervention groups in respect of some valid measurable outcome whilst at the same time ensuring these groups are comparable for any other conceivable influences on outcome. This like with like can be achieved by randomization so long as the groups contain enough subjects. The smaller the number of subjects the more likely might imbalance creep in by the play of chance alone. Small studies run the risk that some factor unknown to the investigator and which correlates to the study outcome could bias the comparison of interventions. Consider this example of a very small randomized study:

Drug A   2 from 20 persons suffer relapse within one year of treatment.

Mean age 45 years, with no person 65 years or older.

Drug B   7 from 20 persons suffer relapse within one year of treatment.

Mean age 55 years, with 5 persons 65 years or older.

Those patients receiving drug A are younger as a group. Suppose Age and outcome are related. In this small experiment an age imbalance in the randomization has occurred by chance.

Although drug A might at first appear better than drug B its favourable standing may only be a consequence of it being taken by younger patients.

And, who can say whether there are other important character imbalances between the two groups particularly in regard to variables which are as yet unknown in their importance and hence not measured for this study. A larger sample size reduces the chances of serious imbalances.

More will be said about sample sizes later. Now we unpeel some of the mystery surrounding randomization. A common method is by putting bits of paper in envelopes, as for example:

Children referred for Speech Therapy are to be randomly allocated either to a clinic-based or to a home-based treatment programme.

Each child attends an initial assessment session at clinic during which baseline (or pre-randomization allocation) data is obtained. These data will determine the eligibility of each child for the study. For suitable children their parents will be asked to give their consent.

Then for each of these children a sealed envelope will be opened and a slip of paper pulled out to reveal one or other of the two treatment programmes allocated for that child.

A pile of sealed envelopes will be prepared in advance of the study, half of which contain a slip of paper with the words *clinic-based* and half with the words *home-based*. From the outside all the envelopes look the same, except for a number on the front indicating the order in which the envelopes are to be opened (first child in study = envelope 1, second child = envelope 2, and so on). The person opening the envelope has no idea what it will reveal.

The envelopes can easily be prepared by the statistician involved.

Suppose in the above example that the age of the child was strongly related to outcome. Then to be more sure of achieving a randomization balance for age the randomization could be done separately for younger and older children. One set of envelopes for those under 3 years and another set for those 3 and over might be used. This is stratified randomization, with the age groups forming the strata. The way in which it is decided what goes into each envelope is illustrated opposite.

Randomization Plan:

ENVELOPE NUMBER	UNDER 3 YEARS	3 YEARS & OVER
1	C	H
2	H	H
3	C	C
4	C	C
5	H	H
6	H	H
7	H	C
8	H	C
9	C	H
10	C	C
11	H	H
ETC	ETC	ETC

C=therapy at clinic, H=therapy at home

The choice of C or H is decided by the toss of a coin, with heads=H and tails=C.

According to this plan two sets of envelopes are to be prepared, one set for the under 3's and another set for those 3 and over. Each set is numbered 1,2,3, etc.

By the envelope method it is also possible to ensure equal numbers in each group. Numbers are 'balanced' by an independent person who keeps the balancing points to him/herself. In the above example both strata were balanced after the first 10 children , ensuring 5 'C' and 5 'H'. Other balancing points could be say 22, 46, 68 at the discretion of the 'independent' person.

Stratified methods are usually employed in smaller studies where there might justifiably be worries about chance imbalances. The ideal however is to aim for large enough sample sizes to make prior stratification unnecessary. Stratification does increase trial administration, and can increase the chance of allocation error (when patients do not receive the treatment to which they have been allocated). Try to avoid more than 2 strata.

There are various ways of deciding what goes into which envelope and indeed there are other methods of allocating in a random manner without envelopes, though envelopes do carry the advantage that the randomization procedure can be prepared well in advance and preferably in secret by someone (perhaps a statistician) who remains independent of the day to day management of trial subjects.

The method of alternation, by which patients are allocated alternatively to treatments, isn't a random process since it is possible to pre-select patients to coincide with the next known alternate treatment. If you know that the next treatment is to be placebo you might be tempted to save dear old Mrs smith until next time and put her onto the drug you have great expectations of. Fully random methods are less easy to tamper with by those people involved in the day to day activities underpinning the study and who may be unaware of the value of random allocation. It is very important that such people don't know what the next allocation will be. To adopt fully random methods is far easier than having to counter criticisms levelled against the method of alternation.

Insist on keeping a simple list of all subjects considered for entry to a study together with either the result of randomization or the reason why randomization didn't occur. For example:

1) Patient's name ....

2A) Patient ineligible because
....

2B) Patient eligible but refused to participate because
....

2C) Patient eligible, strata group ...., randomly allocated to .....
from envelope number ....

```
1) Jo Bloggs
2A)       Child ineligible because of a profound hearing loss requiring special
          educational placement.

1) John Brown
2B)       Child eligible but parents refused to give consent because they didn't
          want their child to be "experimented on".

1) Jim BiLu
2C)       Child eligible, aged under 3 years, randomly allocated to Home
          therapy from envelope number 6.
```

A list like this of all subjects considered will later enable you to give a better, more realistic interpretation of results. It will also help you to guard against sloppiness which could show for example in a suitable child being excluded. If several persons are responsible for administering the entry criteria then this list will provide a check of consistency between them.

Relax the exclusion criteria as much as possible. The more centres, hospitals, practices the better. Include as wide a range of subjects as possible. Too narrow a range and the study loses its external validity, that is you will find it difficult to generalise.

Clinical Trial

Desirable features of a controlled clinical trial are a clearly defined and important study hypothesis, a randomized allocation of patients to treatment, a double-blind assessment of all patients at all times, a large enough sample size to virtually avoid missing any improvements worth knowing about, a minimum of patient withdrawal or non-compliance, an identical management policy for each patient except for the nature of the treatments, and the resources and administration necessary for carrying the plan through.

Administration involves ensuring that the right person is in the right place at the right time to make the right measurement on the right patient, and so on. The random allocation needs careful administration too. A dedicated organised enthusiast is needed to mastermind operations, someone aware of the desirable principles of controlled trials. A well planned study does provide the informed researcher with the confidence of knowing that a well organised study will produce results of clinical value. The prevailing climate for conducting a clinical trial is that there is uncertainty about the effectiveness of a proposed intervention. A clinician firmly of the opinion that drug A is better than drug B is in no strong ethical position to participate in a study in which some of his or her patients may be allocated to drug B. A stance of uncertain neutrality has to be the norm for participating clinicians and those with strong preferences should be discouraged from taking part.

Clearly the time for experimental evaluation of a new drug, treatment or procedure is at the time when it is first being introduced. If a drug is in general use it becomes increasingly difficult to avoid giving it, particularly if no other known therapy exists.

A problem arises when patients fail to complete their prescribed course of treatment. If they are lost to follow-up and excluded from the analysis this could seriously bias the results especially if their reason for dropping out was related to treatment (eg a patient withdraws because of severe mood changes soon after taking the treatment drug). You should always endeavour to continue to observe such patients to the end of the observation period irrespective of any changes to protocol (ie the above patient would still be encouraged to come for assessments after the drug treatment had ceased or had been changed).

If the number of protocol violations are very small then it makes little difference to the overall results. If the numbers are considerable then a trial that began as a neat comparison of treatments would have to be converted into a comparison of the policy of intending to treat one way and the policy of intending to treat in another way. Thus all those initially randomized into the study are included in the analysis to provide a randomized comparison of treatment intentions.

Drug A: 300 pts:
80 withdraw from treatment during study period
220 continue with treatment to end of study period

Drug B: 300 pts:
9 withdraw from treatment during study period
291 continue with treatment to end of study period

The final <u>outcome</u> is relapse within one year of entry to the study. Information is available for all 600 patients.

The randomized "like with like" comparison is of:

<u>Intention to treat with Drug A</u> (300 patients)
VS
<u>Intention to treat with Drug B</u> (300 patients)

It is unreasonable to compare the 220 (Drug A) patients against the 291 (Drug B) patients because it is no longer a comparison of "like with like". Withdrawal bias has eaten more into group A and who knows what imbalances in other characteristics this has introduced.

The bias of non-compliance will often eat into one treatment group more than the other. It follows therefore that all patients entered into a randomized controlled trial should be followed up for the full planned period regardless of any treatment violations, except of course when patients refuse to have anything else to do with the research.

The proportion of eligible patients who consent to randomization will vary according to the nature of the study. For a trial comparing operation and some conservative therapy this proportion might be quite low. There is then a good case to go for a total (eligible) cohort study in which the non-randomized patients can be considered alongside the trial patients who agree to random allocation:

Eligible patients:

Consent	Random Allocation	Follow-up assessments?
YES	OPERATION	YES
YES	CONSERVATIVE THERAPY	YES
NO	NONE	YES

Finally in this section, a flow diagram (see below) is a good way of portraying key aspects of design in both protocols and reports:

Flow diagram for trial of "new" drug vs "usual" drug in new cases of joint pain. Randomization and Drug treatment:

```
    Visit 1                          Visit 2
      |                                |
    Day 0                            Day 28
      |                                |
      |---------------|----------------------|
      | [A]   two "new" tablets each morning |
      |   + one "placebo" tablet 3 times a day|
      |                                | treatment
  Randomization                       | stops
   to A or B                          | after
      |                                | 28 days
      | [B]   one "usual" tablet 3 times a day|
      |     two "placebo" tablets each morning|
      |---------------|----------------------|
```

In group A the placebo tablets are disguised to look, feel and taste the same as the "usual" tablets.

In group B the placebo tablets are disguised to look, feel and taste the same as the "new" tablets.

Thus each patient's combination of tablets look, feel and taste identical.

Flow diagram for trial of "new" drug vs "usual" drug in new cases of joint pain. <u>Data Collection</u>:

```
Visit 1              Visit 2         Questionnaire
   |                    |               by post
 Day 0                Day 28        Day 90   Day 180
   |                    |              |        |
   |                    |              |        |
   |                    |              |        |
Assessments             |              |        |
  before              Blind         Blind    Blind
 randomization      assessments    assessments
   |                    |              |        |
   |                    |              |        |
   |                    |              |        |
Assessment              |              |        |
of eligibility.         |              |        |
Keep Log of all         |              |        |
exclusions,with         |              |        |
reason for exclusion.   |              |        |
   |                    |              |        |
 Clinical            Clinical          |        |
 Examination         Examination       |        |
   |                    |              |        |
Quality of Life    Quality of Life  Quality of life
Questionnaire      Questionnaire    Questionnaire
```

Interactions

The effects of one or more interventions can be studied simultaneously in the same experiment. For example:

---

1) Consider two drugs A and B in the treatment of mild hypertension and suppose that there is no contra-indication to the two drugs being used together:

All eligible patients are randomly assigned to one of four groups (no drug, A only, B only, both A and B).

The effect of A can be estimated by contrasting those two groups using A (A only, A+B) with those two groups not using A (no drug, B only). Likewise the effect of B can be estimated by contrasting groups using B (B only, A+B) with those groups not using B (no drug, A only). This pooling together of groups does make the important assumption that the effects of the two drugs are independent of one another. If there is good reason to suspect an interaction effect (eg effect of A differs according to the presence or absence of B) then the effects of A alone and of B alone can each be separately estimated by comparison with the no drug group. The nature of any interaction can also be studied.

---

2) In general practice which is the best way of encouraging people to attend for preventative screening? Does a simple letter of invitation bear as much fruit as tagging all relevant patient notes and making a verbal invitation when the patient next attends surgery? Is there value in doing both?

Patients are randomly allocated to one of four groups (letter only, tagging of notes only, both methods, neither method).

In this example, cross-contamination between groups could occur and it would be important to ascertain the reasons why people have attended the screening (eg wished to attend because next door neighbour received letter).

Crossover studies

Under certain conditions subjects can be used as their own controls. Each subject receives more than one intervention, with the order of intervention being determined by random allocation:

Consider two different therapeutic diets in patients with long-standing eczema. Each patient would receive both diets, each say of four weeks duration, the patient either being randomly allocated to receive diet A followed by diet B, or to receive diet B followed by diet A. To avoid there being any carry over effect from one therapeutic diet into the next a suitable *washout* period is necessary during which time neither diet is given and patients are encouraged to return to pre-study diets.

Patient outcome during the time on treatment includes a body area affected score, a body itch score and antihistamine consumption.

One advantage of a crossover design follows from the expectation that a comparison of interventions on the same patient will be more precise than a comparison between different patients. By getting more information from each patient the hope is to reduce the total number of patients studied. It generally makes more sense to wish to compare 2 different interventions on the same patient than to compare two different patients. However this type of design has its limitations and would make no sense at all in many situations.

A suitable disease condition is one that displays stability and which doesn't naturally regress nor resolve during the period of study. Also it should be such that if a successful intervention is stopped then the signs and symptoms would reappear.

The crossover design is unsuited to long-term outcomes since the potential gain in sample size would be at the expense of a very long study period.

The number of withdrawals after a study starts should be negligible. A high dropout rate greatly weakens a study especially if dropout is associated with one of the interventions. The comparison of interventions in the second phase would be biased, and for this reason the inclusion in analysis of only those patients who complete both stages is to be discouraged. It may be that only the first phase results are of any scientific value:

Pre-random Allocation	1ST Diet	Patients Left	2ND Diet	Patients Left
N=100	Diet A	76	Diet B	74
		Washout Period		
N=100	Diet B	97	Diet A	87

To compare the remaining 74 and 87 patients is inadvisable since who knows what selective biases have crept into the reckoning.

The only reasonable (and randomized) comparison in the above example is of the intention to treat by diet A (N=100) with the intention to treat by diet B (N=100). All patients are assessed at the end of the first phase regardless of whether they have stopped the therapeutic diet. But this is no more than the randomized clinical trial described earlier.

A serious problem arises if a period-treatment interaction is present, that is if the difference between treatment outcome varies according to the phase of the study. An insufficient washout time between treatments might produce a carryover effect from one treatment to the next. The potential for change on treatment B might thus be affected by a lingering carryover from treatment A. Again, analysis of the first phase results only is recommended:

Baseline Assessment:	Group1 pts	Mean Body Itch Score 70
	Group2 pts	Mean Body Itch Score 70
End of 1ST Phase:	1.Diet A	Mean Body Itch Score 30
	2.Diet B	Mean Body Itch Score 50
End of 2ND Phase:	1.Diet B	Mean Body Itch Score 30
	2.Diet A	Mean Body Itch Score 30

Following baseline assessment patients were randomly allocated to two groups: group 1 to receive diet A then diet B, group 2 to receive diet B then diet A.

There looks to be a carryover effect from phase 1 into phase 2. Perhaps some patients were reluctant to adhere to the second phase diet B after having made good progress with the first phase diet A.

Statistical tests between treatments rely largely on the assumption that there is no period-treatment interaction (ie treatment differences are assumed to be the same for each phase). This assumption itself can be checked by statistical methods, the precision of which depend upon the number of subjects in the study. A satisfactory check would require large numbers of patients since it is based on between subject rather than within subject variability. This negates the advantage of choosing a crossover study in the first place. If evidence of an interaction is found then only the first phase results can be usefully analysed.

So think long and hard if you want to do a crossover study. They may be useful with chronic diseases that remain stable over a long period of time & with palliative care rather than cures. The burden of proof rests on you to demonstrate that the crossover design does have advantages over the more usual and simpler parallel clinical trial design. Previous evidence indicating the absence of carryover effects, low dropout rates, a fairly stable disease process over time, and a relevant short term response would clearly help in this. The potential saving in the number of patients has to be set against the more complicated crossover analysis and higher patient dropout through longer patient involvement. When using a crossover design aim for double-blind conditions and for the same management of each patient as one would in an ordinary randomized controlled trial.

Bias and the control of variables

In case-control, cohort and experimental research it is vitally important to be able to anticipate, recognise, minimise or avoid bias when seeking to compare. The onus is on you to plan to eliminate, and to be seen to have eliminated, all forms of bias as far as is practically possible. Known unavoidable biases should be addressed in your protocol as well when you report your results.

Explanatory variables are variables that might relate to and possibly explain the outcomes of interest. These variables are defined and weaved into the questions and background of the research and highlighted by hypotheses in statements of purpose. In seeking to describe the relationship between an explanatory variable and a study outcome, one has to accept that there may be other extraneous variables that will interfere with this. With a sufficient sample size experimental randomization should minimise such problems by scattering extraneous influences equally amongst the explanatory groups. However, there may still be other biases around which arise systematically from the way subjects are managed during their time in the study:

Explanatory Variable:	Extraneous Variable:	Extraneous Variable:
Type of care	Surgeon	Anaesthesia
Day-case	Surgeon A	Local
Inpatient	Surgeon B	General

A randomized comparison of Day-case and Inpatient cataract surgery would clearly be compromised if all those patients randomly allocated to the Day-case group were operated on by surgeon A and all those allocated to the Inpatient group were operated on by surgeon B. The extraneous disturbing variable is the surgeon, and would represent a bias arising from the way the experiment was organised. The inability to separate this extraneous variable from the explanatory variable (Type of Care) means that an independent assessment of the methods of care on trial is impossible. One solution to this problem would be to have the randomization allocation (as Day-case or Inpatient) stratified by surgeon.

A similar problem might occur in the above example if the day-case operations were to be done under local anaesthesia whilst inpatient operations were to be done under general anaesthesia. Again stratification is one answer. However, if the type of anaesthesia is regarded as an integral part of the management of the patient then it becomes an integral part of the explanatory variable, that is of day-case or inpatient care.

Another example is the smoking status of patients in a study evaluating the usefulness of oxygen cylinder therapy for persons suffering severe respiratory problems:

O_2 Cylinder therapy	- Smokers
	- Non-Smokers
NO O_2 Cylinder therapy	- Smokers
	- Non-Smokers

It could be argued that because of the risks of explosion those patients receiving oxygen therapy have a greater incentive to cut down or to stop smoking. Thus the value of oxygen therapy as measured by changes in respiratory function is confounded with changes in smoking habit. One possible solution would be to only include patients into the study if they had definitely given up smoking. Another would be to stratify any analyses by smoking habit.

The problem with non-experimental comparison studies is that there may well be important extraneous variables that remain unidentified. (At least with randomization you can feel reasonably secure that any unidentified influences will affect each group to a similar extent). If extraneous variables can be identified then one should try to measure them. At least then results can be stratified by such variables.

Another technique of control involves *matching* to ensure a similarity in the distribution of values for certain variables within comparison groups. There is however a limit on the number of variables you can usefully match on, and matching does tend to be wasteful of resources.

Alternatively there is *restricted selection* by which you would restrict the range that important extraneous variables take and thus obtain a greater purity or homogeneity in the selected sample. Wishing to exclude certain subject subgroups reflects concern about the relationship with the study outcomes. If smoking were the offending variable, as in the O_2 example above then the research might be focused entirely on non-smokers. The great danger of excluding one subgroup after another is that it makes the focus of the research narrow and limits generalisation.

In trying to establish causality the chance you always take with an observational study is that alternative explanations are possible. Any observed relationship between a proposed explanatory variable and an outcome variable may or may not be causal. In general assume not and then look for alternative explanations and try to control for these. Several observational studies using different controlling mechanisms, and which produce similar correlations (eg as with smoking and respiratory disease) provide a more convincing argument than any single isolated study.

An experiment allows greater control of unwanted influences but again the repeated evidence from several studies is stronger than from a single study. The meta-analyses that exist try to bring together from a variety of published sources (and unpublished if possible to reduce positive publication bias) an accumulation of information relating to similar hypotheses.

The rational of the meta-analysis approach is that treatment effects observed in different trials will tend to go in the same direction. Methods have developed in an attempt to introduce rigour to the task of drawing a consensus from many small and medium sized trials each addressing a closely related question. Certain trials will be methodologically stronger than others, and the populations studied might differ quite considerably. Very large trials may be required to detect very small but yet important clinical benefits and in the absence of these a meta-analysis does at least include a large number of patients, be they from a number of different trials. The meta-analysis approach shouldn't be seen as a substitute for planning large studies nor should it be seen as an excuse for having done a small study.

Further reading (See Chapter 9 for full list of references):

Ref 1 (chpt 20, 21, 22)
Ref 2 (chpt 21, 22, 24, 25)
Ref 3 (chpt 8, 9, 10, 11, 12)
Ref 6 (p9-15, p37-41, p47-63)
Ref's 5, 8, 25, 27, 29, 31, 34, 35, 36,

3. ETHICAL ISSUES

You should by now have a reasonable idea of the type of study you will do. In this chapter we reflect upon the ethics of doing research. Many of the decisions you will make about design, administration and analysis do carry ethical implications. As you read through this chapter you may be surprised at the number of moral issues that can arise from doing research. So, as you read, make a note of anything that worries you about your research plans. Be prepared to adjust your plans accordingly.

Choosing research to do

Finding funds for research is a big problem and the total amount of funds available defines a ceiling to the amount of research that can take place. The holders of purse-strings obviously have a large say in what topics are researched. The main funding bodies are the state (especially through the universities, the research councils, and the department of health), industry (especially pharmaceutical and electronics), and charities and trusts. The prestigious awards and professional status all lean towards technological innovation and the frontiers of biomedical research. Research/audit into the process of care and of different ways of doing what is already being done appears to come a poor second particularly in professional status.

How rational is the balance in medical research? What influences and pressures (commercial, political, media, professional peers, general public) are there as to what research gets done and where are the gaps? How do you and your research ideas fit into the general scheme of things?

Why would you choose to do a particular piece of research? Might it arise directly from your professional activities? Perhaps you wish to contribute to the general accumulation of knowledge. Maybe it is a requirement for higher qualification. Perhaps the research is likely to come up with newsworthy results. You may feel forced into it by your professional superiors. It could be that you really do need the job and would greatly appreciate the money that goes with the research.

Perhaps the far-flung trails of the research conferences are ones you wish to tread. Probably it's a combination of these. The aim of this section is not to be rude but for us all to simply and honestly explore our own reasons for undertaking the research we do. Do we really feel under pressure to bolster our curriculum vitaes and are we prepared to sacrifice quality for quantity in our efforts for quick results? Would we apply for a research project post that we knew was funded by money from certain industries, or by a company with known investments in certain parts of the world? Would we agree to do research without a clear prior statement that any results from it could be submitted for publication?

What criteria might we apply when approached to collaborate in a study being co-ordinated by someone else? A sound study design should be one priority and this involves a critical approach to the research methodology, as much as if you were designing it yourself. Insist on seeing a detailed protocol.

Ethical considerations for a research project

In general bad research methods constitute bad ethics. At worst the study conclusions might simply be wrong and mislead others into taking inappropriate actions. At best the bad methods will be seen for what they are and will encourage better research.

Protocol review

Peer review should draw attention to protocols and reports that are incomplete or out of balance. The consequences of slipping through the net include the use of scarce resources better employed elsewhere and the misleading representation of research within the context of other relevant work.

Background and Literature Review

This should be as balanced and complete an account of the state of knowledge. Do not knowingly present a one-sided and self-supporting account.

An inadequate review of literature could lead to unnecessary duplication of work already done elsewhere.

Populations and Samples

Inappropriate choices could seriously hinder the usefulness of study results. Be aware of the differences between target and study populations and of the problems when generalising from convenience samples.

Informed consent

There is *consent* and there is *informed consent*. By informed consent is meant enough information about the study being given in a way that is clearly understandable to the subject concerned whilst leaving that individual the freedom to choose.

What is meant by *enough* information? The list is endless:- nature and purpose of study, length of participation required, the methods and procedures by which data is collected, the potential harms, side-effects and discomforts reasonably to be expected from participation and how any injuries would be treated if need be, the potential benefits to the subject and from the study as a whole, the option to withdraw from the study at any time without the need to give any explanation, security and confidentiality of personal data. If the study is a randomized clinical trial then other information is required:-- the fact that the subject would be taking part in an experiment, a description of the interventions on trial, the fact that the efficacy of one intervention over any of the others had not been established and the fact that the intervention for the subject would be decided by a process of random allocation.

The freedom to choose requires that the subject feels free to choose. One difficulty is that patients who rely heavily on the advice of their doctors, especially when very ill, feel submissive and vulnerable and may sense that refusal would later be punished. Patient vulnerability can easily be taken advantage of.

The nature of informed consent implies that you should obtain a freely given consent before attempting any of the planned protocol measurements with the subject. The big worry is that the giving of a great deal of information could confuse, overwhelm, upset, or anger a large number of subjects who consequently would refuse to take part. Such non-response could seriously affect the credibility of results. In certain studies full or even partial disclosure could mean giving unwanted, distressful information to patients about their condition, methods of treatment, and of likely prognosis. In others it may be felt that the professional-patient relationship would be undermined. In certain randomized controlled trials full disclosure might work against desirable design features of blinding techniques, dummy placebo treatments and the randomization itself. Imagine yourself as a very frail elderly person being told about the uncertainty of the relative effectiveness of two types of lens implantation, that you would be randomly allocated from an envelope at the time of cataract surgery to receive one or other type, and that for reasons of scientific validity about obtaining honest unbiased measurements from you after surgery you would not be told whether you had had the new or the old type of lens. Perhaps it wouldn't be put quite like this though this is what it might sound like.

It is difficult to envisage the full implications of freely given informed consent being possible in every research project though that should be the aim. One has to give individual rights as much attention as possible without destroying the validity of the study and the onus should be on the investigator to demonstrate in the protocol that informing the subject would invalidate the research. Inconvenience is an unreasonable excuse.

If contact with the subject is solely through a postal questionnaire survey then a covering letter of invitation should also include details such as where their name and address came from, what the study is about, that their data will be treated in confidence, that they can refuse to participate and if they do participate they can refuse to answer particular questions if they so wish. If there is no underlying professional-subject relationship then subjects in a community survey can simply and freely decline to take part by simply not replying. Few people given such information about an important health survey would be die-hard non-responders, though they may need to be sent a reminder or two. If there is an underlying doctor-patient relationship then striving for freely given consent would involve trying to remove any fears about the future harmony of that relationship.

Face to face contact raises other problems. The desire to obtain a good response could lead to verbal over-persuasion. Freely given consent is compounded both by location of interview (at home, hospital or clinic) and by the relationship to the interviewer (as doctor, consultant, nurse, layperson).

Consent may be written or verbal. A written consent document should ideally include the requirements as laid out above. Minors and persons with legal guardians cannot give consent and in these cases parents or guardians must be approached.

Ethical committees

It is in experimental studies that ethical concerns about consent are voiced most strongly. The experimental horrors of world war two led to the development of the Nuremburg Code which set out guide-lines to protect human rights in research. The Helsinki Code (as adopted by the 18th world assembly in 1964 and revised by the 29th in 1975 and the 35th in 1983) now stands as a guide to physicians in biomedical research involving human subjects. On the issue of informed consent the guide-lines both stress the need for adequately informed consent whilst accepting that there will be occasions where this is impossible.

On the one hand we have "In any research on human beings, each potential subject must be adequately informed of the aims, methods, anticipated benefits and potential hazards of the study and the discomfort it may entail." On the other hand "If the physician considers it essential not to obtain informed consent the specific reasons for this proposal should be stated in the experimental protocol for transmission to the independent committee". One of the basic principles of the code was that "The design and performance of each experimental procedure involving human subjects should be clearly formulated in an experimental protocol which should be transmitted to a specially appointed independent committee for consideration, comment and guidance". Hence the submission in this country of study protocols for ethical approval. In a multi-centre study each centre has to seek approval from its own local ethical committee.

Although there is no generally agreed rule on when to seek ethical approval many would argue that any research involving human subjects should require ethical approval. Ethical committee responsibilities particularly concern the misuse of patients, healthy volunteers, animals and other resources. Given that bad design is bad ethics then sub-standard research constitutes a misuse of resources. It could be argued that in the interests of better research all study protocols should be submitted for ethical approval and that ethical committees should broaden their scope of reference.

Variables

The most important variables in any research should be supported by evidence of reliability and validity. Newly developed ways of assessment particularly require confirmation since people could otherwise be misled into assuming the data and conclusions presented are valid.

Sample size

A problem with small studies is that their results may be consistent with a wide range of conclusions. A small clinical trial runs the danger of failing to demonstrate important improvements except perhaps for absolutely massive effects. There is an ethical obligation to seek to enrol enough subjects so as to have a good chance of addressing the research hypotheses. Either too few or too many patients represents a misuse of resources. Justifications of sample size for any kind of study should be presented both in the protocol design and in any subsequent reports.

Pilot study

A research protocol should describe plans for a pilot or dummy run so as to test out the data collection methods being used, the organisational procedures, the randomization scheme, and so forth. To omit this stage could lead to fatal problems being discovered much later on in the day and completely undermine the analysis and interpretation of results, as well as waste the resources committed to that point. So please think seriously about doing a pilot study to iron out any unforeseen problems early on and before you commit the majority of your resources.

Other issues of design

Failure to randomize (eg to use alternation) or to adopt double or single-blind techniques when they are possible makes a controlled trial less acceptable than it need be. Resources would have been better employed in a study with these features.

A placebo or dummy treatment is clearly unethical when there is a known effective treatment already in existence.

Allow a study to run its planned course if at all possible. The decision to terminate a study shouldn't be made prematurely on the basis of early promising trends which fail to satisfy statistical considerations. Other people won't be sufficiently convinced and may set up their own studies, thereby increasing the overall resources required to provide an answer to your question.

Interim analyses where appropriate would allow an earlier termination of a trial if any differences between interventions are greater than initially anticipated. Seek statistical advice on this matter.

Analysis, presentation and interpretation

By ensuring that a numerical serial number, instead of the name and address of a subject, enters a computer system then the only way to establish the full identity of that subject is by cross-referencing between computer and manually held lists. Confidentiality then lies in keeping manual lists away from prying eyes.

When presenting results the disclosure of subject identity is generally regarded as unethical. Participating centres and individuals doing the research are generally happy to be identified, but what of listing those centres or individual professionals who were approached but refused to take part? Such information could help in the general applicability of results. What of the ethics of revealing evidence of professional ill-treatment, negligence or incompetence that plays an important part in explaining the results?

The misuse of statistical methods has ethical implications since at the very worst the interpretation from the results could be completely wrong. Even if the methods are correct the interpretation could still be wrong. There is also an ethical obligation to publish the results of one's research irrespective of the result. Not to seek to do so leads to a bias in the type of reports submitted for publication. Journals also have an ethical responsibility to insist on and accept only good quality research.

Further reading (See Chapter 9 for full list of references):

Ref 1 (p203-8, p232-8)
Ref 3 (p271-2)
Ref 5 (p100-9)
Ref's 8, 17, 37, 40

4. SAMPLING METHODS

This chapter looks at a variety of ways in which samples can be chosen from a population. Ultimately you will be hoping that the subjects you study are representative in some meaningful way of the population to which you wish to generalise. You have to be careful to use the resources at your disposal to maximum effect, to achieve a better representation. There will be situations when your ways of choosing a sample are limited and indeed even your best method may have its problems. This chapter will help you get the best from your sampling and encourage you to recognise the strengths and weaknesses of the various options open to you.

The problems of generalising from sample to study population and then to target population have already been discussed in chapters 1 and 2. The gap between study and target populations has to be considered in terms of systematic non-random error, or bias. The gap between sample and study population is a combination of random and non-random error.

Populations:	
Target:	UK adults
Study:	Adults registered with one Health Practice in central Manchester.
Sample:	1 in 10 random sample from list of study population. 70% of those selected agree to take part.

Random or probability sampling implies that for each member of the study population it is possible to compute the chance (or probability) of being chosen in the sample. Such sampling requires that each member of the population is known.

Random sampling isn't an automatic guarantee of representativeness since there is always a chance that an unlikely sample will be produced by the random process, as in the next example:

Study Population: boys and girls aged 11-16 attending schools in your town. Suppose there are 1200 boys and 1200 girls. All children are identified and given a study number from 1 to 2400.

Sample 1: random sample of 1 in 100 children. Thus 24 of the 2400 numbers were selected using a random method, giving: *15 boys and 9 girls*

Sample 2: random sample of 1 in 10 Children. Thus 240 of the 2400 numbers were selected giving: *125 boys and 115 girls*

Random sampling errors can be controlled by ensuring enough subjects are taken into the sample, as in the above where a better ratio of boys to girls is achieved.

It is random sampling that provides the bridge between the statistical analysis of sample data and the study population. Random sampling allows for an unbiased estimation of summary parameters such as means or percentages. In the absence of random sampling then systematic bias could easily (and unknowingly) creep into the sample and parameter estimates would then be biased.

Sampling Frames

Having identified a target population you need to gain access to a suitable sampling frame. An ideal sampling frame is a list which identifies each and every member of that population. If a single list is forthcoming then random sampling from it is straightforward.

Examples of sampling frames include electoral roll lists, school lists, general practice registrations, FPC lists, telephone books, occupational registers, computer pay-roll lists, armed forces service numbers, birth registers and computerised lists of patients admitted to hospital.

Whether you find a particular sampling frame useful will depend on its accuracy, its representativeness of the target population, and its convenience. The task of drawing up a single list of population members for random sampling can be daunting (eg a list of all schoolchildren attending schools in the local authority) or practically impossible (eg child solvent abusers). Adopting a more convenient method of sampling (eg choosing a small

number of schools and then choosing a random sample of children from within each selected school) would save time, money and resources generally. Such savings have to be balanced against the purpose of the research and most especially the representativeness of the resulting sample.

A sampling frame might in error contain some members more than once, either as an obvious duplication or less obviously as a similar but misspelt surname. Lists might be out of date.

Since the composition of a sampling frame can change with time, such as with a GP Practice list, then it is necessary to choose some relevant starting point and to use the list that represents the population at that time point:

> In a general practice prevalence survey of emphysema a list known to be accurate at the beginning of the study is used. Every person selected will be visited at home. The time taken to visit everyone on the list will be considerable, during which period new patients enter the practice and some patients die or migrate.

Having defined a list at the beginning of a study the task of the researcher is to try and account for every person sampled from that list. Newcomers into a general practice would be excluded from the study list though they might possibly be considered as an additional group.

Non-Probability sampling

Random sampling methods should be employed wherever appropriate and it is an inferior design that proposes to do otherwise. Making a list of all members of the relevant population is often impossible or is at best highly impracticable. However, in very exploratory research it may well be that a convenience population ideally suits the purpose of the study, as in a pilot study to test out the wording and administration of a questionnaire or interview. Examples of populations in which a compilation of a list of members would be difficult include women in menopause, alcoholics, pipe smokers, hard drug addicts, and many diseases. For certain groups registers do exist, eg local psychiatric registers, register of children with phenylketenuria, people with Raynaud's disease. Problems of accuracy and representativeness apply to registers as much as with any other list.

Subjects who respond to a newspaper advertisement for research volunteers form a *convenience sample*, as do healthy normal hospital volunteers. Many samples in medical research are convenient because of the easy presentation of patients for treatment. Those who remain undiagnosed, who fail to present, or who don't get referred are by default excluded. How representative are such convenience patients of all those with the disease in question?

A method that leaves the choice of subject to the eye of the researcher won't be random. The bias may well remain unknown both in type and degree. As an interviewer on the streets you might unconsciously, even deliberately, choose those faces that look as though they would like to be interviewed. We can guess then that your sample will be biased towards friendly looking faces. You may deny this but what evidence is there one way or the other? Interviewers who are told to conduct a certain number of house-call interviews are likely to chase those easiest to reach, for example those who happen to be at home when called upon.

You have most likely been stopped on the street at some time, and questioned about your consumption habits or political leanings by someone collecting to a predetermined quota. A *quota sample* based on five age groups and on sex would mean that the interviewer has to recruit a pre-specified number of interviewees in each of 10 age-sex categories. This approach though giving the sample a logical balance in age and sex characteristics similar to the local population does conceal bias arising from face-to-face methods of selection and from non-response. Quota sampling fails to force researchers to think about minimising non-response, and if non-response goes unrecorded this will inevitably weaken a study.

Network sampling uses human social networks to generate a sample by encouraging contact along network channels. Finding one person with characteristics relevant for study leads to contact with friends and acquaintances of that person who also have similar characteristics. The approach to friends and acquaintances is best made by those persons already in the study. Network sampling might help in circumstances when the principle characteristics under study are ones which are generally devalued in society at large or are ones for which direct revelation to strangers is unlikely.

In summary you should aim at getting a large enough random sample from a suitable sampling frame. This will mean that your results can be more meaningfully interpreted. Write any compromises you have to make from this sampling ideal into your protocol and explain why you have decided to choose a more convenient approach to sampling. Discuss the consequences of doing so.

Simple random sampling

Simple random sampling means that each person in the population has an equal, and known, chance of being selected. If all these people can be identified, they can each be given a number (1,2,3 and so on) and a simple random sample can be drawn. Find a method to generate random numbers, such as a calculator with a random number generating function, or random number tables (which are merely page upon page of digits, literally generated at random).

If your computer holds all the names you might be able to use it (or rather its software) to generate a random sample of names. Or alternatively you could write every name on a bit of paper (a computer might produce labels of the same size for you) and drop these into a large bag, get several people to thoroughly shuffle and shake the bag, and then get someone else to draw out the required number of names. This last method is least favoured since randomness depends on how well the bag is shaken. For example if names are prepared alphabetically, the bag is poorly shaken, and names are consistently drawn from the top then an alphabetical bias may result. This may result in an under or over representation of certain cultural groups in the sample.

Simple random sampling doesn't necessarily mean you will end up with a simple random sample. If only 25% of those selected through simple random sampling bother to complete and return your questionnaire then it cannot be said that these responders form a random sample from the population.

Systematic sampling

The use of simple random sampling requires that population members be identified and listed. If a general practice has a computerised registration system then simple random sampling is possible from computer software permitting the random output of names. Otherwise the preparation of a patient list from patient records in practice envelopes is an awesome task. However, so long as the total practice size is known, if only approximately, then there is the option of taking a systematic sample, a method that avoids most of the drudgery.

Imagine a group practice of about 16000 patients half of whom are male. Suppose a sample of 400 males is to be chosen. The sampling fraction is 400 from 8000, or about 1 in 20 males.

To carry out a systematic sample first choose a number at random between 1 and 20 by some simple random process. Having done this (suppose 15 was selected at random) then work through all the folders in a systematic order and select every 20th person (records 15, 35, 55, 75, 95, 115, and so on).

The important thing is to scan through all records, and to include each record only once. The order of doing so is less important.

Although the interest is in sampling males the scanning of all records will include females as well. This is inevitable without having to do the vastly greater chore of separating out male from female records in the first place. The female records can be put straight back into the filing system from whence they were momentarily plucked. In all about 800 patient files will have been looked at, half male and half female.

The systematic sample is still a random sample if at the outset all persons have an equal chance of appearing in the sample. The random choice of the first person in the list however determines those who make up the remainder of the sample and thus only a small number of samples (20 in the example given) are possible.

There are situations in which the representativeness of a systematic sample is doubtful. If there is evidence of cyclical patterns within the ordering then fixed interval sampling might regularly over-sample a small part of the cycle. A systematic sample of patients from an operation list or from an hospital

admissions list may unwittingly coincide with an underlying cycle and may thereby over-represent certain days of the week. Any part-time researcher working one or two fixed days a week could face a similar problem if the case-mix is expected to vary throughout the week.

To obtain a representative sample of patients seen in a hospital accident and emergency unit during a 12 month period a 1 in 7 systematic sample of days is undesirable since the same day of the week is always selected. A better way would be to select a day at random from each week. It would be more representative to consider time in seven week blocks and to randomly select the research day for each of the 7 weeks within a block. This could be done to ensure that each day of the week appeared only once during every 7 week period.

Stratified sampling

It can be advantageous to subdivide, or stratify, a population into well defined subgroups (strata) and then to draw a random sample from within each subgroup. For example:

1 in 5 sample of children attending school A
1 in 5 sample of children attending school B
1 in 5 sample of children attending school C

This example shows three strata with a uniform random sampling fraction of 1 in 5 children applying within each stratum. With stratification the balance between the three schools in the combined sample is thus guaranteed to be the same as for all children attending the three schools. This balance cannot be guaranteed if a simple random sample is taken from a single list of all the children.

Consider a survey of the dental health of children. In the ten schools of a locality 1000 children are listed as eligible for study. The intention is to study 200 of these children:

		STRATIFIED	SIMPLE
		1 in 5 random sample from each school	**1 in 5 random sample from 1000 children**
	Total Number of children	Number of children in each sample	Number of children in sample
School A	100	1 in 5 = 20	18
School B	50	1 in 5 = 10	12
School C	200	1 in 5 = 40	35
School D	100	1 in 5 = 20	22
School E	100	1 in 5 = 20	17
School F	110	1 in 5 = 22	25
School G	80	1 in 5 = 16	16
School H	120	1 in 5 = 24	30
School I	90	1 in 5 = 18	20
School J	50	1 in 5 = 10	5

For Simple random sampling all 1000 children are listed, each allocated a number from 1 to 1000 and a sample of 200 chosen.

For stratified sampling a separate list for each school is compiled, each child being allocated a number from 1 to N where N is the number of children in the school. A 1 in 5 simple random sample is then taken from each school.

Suppose the type of school attended is thought to be an important variable in the research. Certain schools might be progressive in their attitude to dental education whereas others may lag behind. Children at one school might come from family backgrounds vastly different to those of children at another school. To best gain an overall picture of dental problems faced by children at school in the locality the sample should be balanced by school in the same proportions as in the study population.

Although the same number of children are selected (ie 200) the overall balance between schools is maintained through stratification but is diluted by simple random sampling that ignores the strata.

Stratification with uniform sampling almost always increases the precision of results over that to be achieved through simple random sampling. The more important the differences between the strata, as far as your research is concerned, the greater the potential gain in precision to be achieved by stratification. Since you can be sure of gaining something in accuracy from stratification you should try and do this whenever possible. For schools above you can substitute hospitals, clinics, general practices or whatever. Whenever you sample patients from more than one important source don't combine the lists into one. Instead, take a random sample from each source using the same sampling fraction.

The choice of strata depends to a large extent on personal judgement. In the previous example the sampling was stratified by school. It could also have been stratified by sex. If sex was thought to be related to the outcomes of the study then stratification by boy and by girl would also have been appropriate. In general you are limited to those variables, such as age and sex, that are known for each member of the sampling frame at the time you sample from it. Some sampling frames, especially computerised systems, do allow for access to other information, for example a hospital maternity computer system providing a list of mothers stratified by age, gestation and birth outcome.

If you know that one or more strata is considerably more variable (in the outcome you wish to measure) than others then it would pay you to over-sample from these, that is you can use a higher sampling fraction in these strata. The aim of over-sampling is to increase the chance of obtaining a more representative sample from the more highly variable groups. However if you do vary the sampling fraction from one stratum to another then you need to take account of this in analysis should you wish to combine the strata together to obtain overall results.

You can also use over-sampling to give you similarly sized samples in comparative studies. For example, the vast majority of preventative screening tests for a certain disease will turn out to be negative. A few will be positive and some may be borderline. Suppose a population of 10000 women are tested during the year and that 2% are classed as positive, 4% are classed as borderline and the remaining 94% are classed as negative. Imagine a study to investigate the way women feel about the screening procedure and how they feel the service could be improved. The test result could well be an important influence in this and it is decided to compare the three groups in data obtained from an in-depth interview:

Test Result	Number of Women	Sampling Fraction	Sample Size
Positive	200	1 in 1	200
Borderline	400	1 in 2	200
Negative	9400	1 in 47	200

Differing sampling fractions are used to give three groups of the same sample size (of 200), enabling separate estimates within each group, and comparisons between groups.

Suppose 20%(40) of the test positive women, 25%(50) of the test borderline women, and 30%(60) of the test negative women were dissatisfied in some way with the screening procedure. An estimate of the level of dissatisfaction for the whole screening population is possible so long as the different sampling fractions are allowed for:

Test Result	Number of Women	Sampling Fraction	Sample Size	Sample Number Dissatisfied	Screening Population Dissatisfied (Projection)
Positive	200	1 in 1	200	40 = 20%	20% = 40
Borderline	400	1 in 2	200	50 = 25%	25% = 100
Negative	9400	1 in 47	200	60 = 30%	30% = 2820

The dissatisfaction rates found in each of the three samples are applied to the total number of women in each of the three populations. Thus a total projected number of women likely to be dissatisfied in some way is 40 + 100 + 2820, ie 2960 out of 10000 women. So, the best estimate of dissatisfaction in the whole of the screened population is 29.6%.

Different sampling fractions within strata allow adequate comparisons to be made with the most economical use of resources.

Cluster Sampling

Clusters are like strata in that both comprise members of a defined study population. However there are differences in the way samples are chosen. The unit of sampling is the group of cluster members rather than the individual member. For example:

Consider the whole of the adult population in the UK that are registered with general practitioners. This population is subdivided, or stratified by single doctor or by group practice. A single list of practices is compiled.

Cluster sampling: a simple random sample of 10 practices is chosen. All adults in each chosen practice are in the study sample.

Another example is a simple random sample of 20 schools (clusters) from a nation-wide list of schools. Every child attending these 20 schools takes part in the study.

Clustering, as its name implies, is often based on closeness of some kind and tends to lead to members of a cluster being somewhat alike. One cluster (patients at one hospital) may be quite different from another cluster (patients at another hospital) in characteristics (eg case-mix) relevant to the main questions under study. When contemplating cluster sampling always think about the representativeness of the resulting sample.

Ideally, clusters should differ as little as possible between themselves in respect of characteristics important to your research. If the population members were scattered at random between the clusters then cluster sampling would be both convenient and representative. The closeness within clusters is often referred to as homogeneity. The greater the segregation of a population into separate clusters the greater is the homogeneity within the cluster.

Cluster sampling is usually chosen for reasons of convenience and expense. Physical closeness of samples cuts down interviewer travel and time, reduces the number of contacts needed (eg permission of a few rather than all clinics or schools) and the administrative effort involved. However it should always be accepted that cluster sampling is likely to lead to some loss in precision of results. Avoid cluster sampling unless there really is no better alternative.

If the number of clusters to be studied is small then a subjective selection might actually better serve the aims of the study than random selection. In this way clusters could be chosen to maximise known differences between clusters. For example:

In one district a small number of child health clinics might be chosen to provide mothers for interview. Given that there are only a few clinics to choose from, a subjective selection would best reflect and maximise known differences in approach to preventative health care.

Multi-Stage Sampling

Multi-stage sampling can combine cluster, stratification and simple random sampling methods. For example a simple random sample of 5 hospitals (clusters) is chosen from within each Regional Health Authority (strata). From each selected cluster a simple random sample of 10 consultants is chosen. This gives a sample of over 500 consultants to whom a questionnaire is to be sent.

For the final sample to be representative of consultants over the whole country it is better to have a large number of hospitals selected and a low sampling fraction within each hospital rather than a small number of hospitals and a high sampling fraction within each hospital. Thus a simple random sample of 10 hospitals from each Region and then a simple random sample of 5 consultants from each hospital would give a better nation-wide representation.

Type of study and sampling methods

Many samples in hospital-based research are chosen for convenience because of the easy availability of patients. Patients become known sequentially as they appear. A longitudinal case-series study to follow patients suffering from subarachnoid haemorrhage and admitted to one neurosurgical unit is an example. If we consider all neurosurgical centres then this single-centre convenience sample is very much like a single cluster. In generalising results from one centre the variation between centres is important. It is clearly more representative of all patients (present and future untreated) to include a greater number of neurosurgical centres rather than perhaps concentrate upon one especially renowned centre of excellence.

Randomized clinical trials often recruit easily accessible subjects presenting at a single treatment centre. One alternative would be to ring up all treatment centres and compile a current list of all patients in the country who satisfy the entry criteria and then to choose a random sample from this list. The more usual (and realistic) approach is either a single-centre (cluster) or multi-centre (several clusters) study. The choice of cluster or clusters may limit the desired generalisation to all clusters, since the choice is unlikely to be random. For any convenience sample so obtained the subsequent random allocation procedure of a clinical trial does however ensure a randomness within the study that allows meaningful statistical comparison of the clinical interventions on trial, at least for the cluster population(s) involved.

Hospital volunteers are often enrolled as *normals* to establish normal ranges, a range of values expected of some variable in the general population. Sometimes a cluster of staff members, sometimes relatives of patients, or sometimes other patients attending for unrelated problems are taken to represent the public at large. The relevance of such *normals* should be questioned. The self-selection of the population in its approach to doctors may lead to considerable bias, as may the sharing of family genes. Certain types of individual may be inaccessible except through a random sample from a community-based sampling frame.

Likewise the controls in a case-control study need to be carefully chosen. A hospital drawn control group may or may not be appropriate to the research. The problem with a community control group is non-response, but efforts to overcome this are well worth it. The use of invasive techniques in research does limit the possibilities for obtaining control subjects, and the enrolment of staff volunteers and patients with other diseases undergoing such invasive procedures may be the only realistic options. Whatever the options available the effects of clustering should never be ignored.

Non-sampling errors

Sampling errors are those that can leave you with a sample that is unrepresentative. These may either be random (eg chance variations in small samples) or non-random (eg selection bias in cluster samples).

Non-sampling errors include errors in taking measurements, in observation or interview, in a badly designed questionnaire, in non-response and in miscoding & mispunching data for computer analysis. Coding and punching errors might tend to cancel out in the long run but this can be by no means be taken as certain and a large error rate in this respect merely represents sloppiness and fails to instil confidence in the study as a whole. Errors in measurement may result from inexperience and from systematic differences between people doing the measuring. Non-sampling error can be reduced by improving the precision of the methods of measurement, by encouraging willing participation, and by improving data collection and processing. A pilot study helps to iron out such difficulties.

Aim at controlling for all types of error. However, it is wasteful to spend huge sums of money in order to obtain a large random sample if substantial non-sampling errors are allowed to remain. Equally well it may be fruitless to spend time perfecting elaborate techniques and procedures if it proves impossible to raise a sufficiently representative sample.

Further reading (See Chapter 9 for full list of references):

Ref 1 (chpt 2, 3)
Ref 2 (chpt 23)
Ref 17, 33

5. DATA MEASUREMENT & COLLECTION

This chapter gets you to look critically at the data you want to collect. You can waste a lot of time and energy by failing to give enough thought to the measurement of variables that are crucial to your study. How will you go about getting reliable and valid information? This chapter explores reliability and validity in a practical way and also explains why it is important to give a lot of thought to the wording of questions, to the layout of record forms and the piloting of the data collection procedure. As part of your protocol you should describe your main variables and say how the data will be collected. Also you should give evidence of reliability and validity, and include your data record forms.

You may be tempted to try and collect as much information as possible, just in case it turns out to be useful. Such logic may seem reasonable but the problem is that data of marginal worth will detract from the collection of essential data. By doing so you may also limit the number of subjects you have time to study. To drown in a sea full of data is a sad end to your enthusiasm.

Which variables

List those variables that are essential to your study. Then list any other variables of minor interest. For each variable describe the amount of detail required and ask whether it is really needed. You may find that asking what, why, when, how, where and who will help you find the required detail, as in this example:

What is the amount of undiagnosed hypertension in a population aged 45 and over and within one large general practice? Those already known to have hypertension, controlled or otherwise, are to be excluded from study. Letters of invitation to screening are to be sent to a random sample from the rest.

WHAT		
	Variable	: BLOOD PRESSURE
	Values Variable takes	: Systolic, Diastolic
		: mm Hg
		: Hypert've, Borderline, Normal

WHY   Essential in any study of hypertension

WHEN		
	Historical	: from GP notes.
	Current	: at screening sessions 2 weeks apart and later at GP surgery if necessary.

HOW		
	Historical	: clerical extraction of data from notes.
	Current	: sphygomanometer.

WHERE

     Practice Premises
     ? Home if no-response to invitation for screening

WHO		
	Practice Nurse	: all invited patients.
	GP	: pts with consistently high pressures as measured by practice nurse.

VALIDITY

     ? Anxiety, pain, full bladder, constricting clothing, cold, place (clinic vs home).

RELIABILITY

     ? Certain equipment requires special training.
     ? Idiosyncratic rounding up or down.

COMMENTS ARISING:

1. Need to define *hypertensive*, *borderline*, and *normal*.
2. How will patients with raised blood pressures be managed ? At which stage does advice give way to drug therapy?
3. How can those failing to respond to invitation be chased up without unnecessary aggravation ? On the other hand if they are not chased then resulting study might either under or over estimate the amount of undiagnosed hypertension.
4. It appears to be convention to seek 3 consistently high readings on separate occasions. This is because in a group of people found to have raised blood pressure on one occasion, a proportion will be found with acceptable lower levels on a second occasion, and a smaller such proportion on a third occasion.

Which variables do you want in your study and why? Justify the inclusion of each. What comments or questions do they raise in the way your study should be organised? Considering each variable in this way will concentrate your mind on to the implications for design.

Some variables that are always worth recording often get ignored. These relate to refusal or non-response. People who refuse to take part in a study, or who later drop out are likely to be different in key aspects to those who do participate in full. Record the reasons for refusal and withdrawal whenever possible. Such data can be thrown into the melting pot to enable more meaningful conclusions to be drawn from the study:

Imagine a multi-clinic survey of mother's attitudes to child health care facilities.

How many clinics were asked to take part in the study? What were the criteria for deciding whether to ask?

Of those clinics asked how many refused to take part and what were the reasons for refusing?

How many mothers attending the participating centres were asked to take part? How many were excluded as unsuitable and why?

Of those mothers considered suitable for the study how many refused to take part and for what reasons? How many subsequently dropped out or refused to answer specific questions, and why?

Answers to such questions have a bearing on the way sample results are interpreted. Such information will help any reader of your work to visualise the groups of subjects actually studied. You need however to collect the information.

In a clinical trial collect as much as possible before randomization and as little as necessary afterwards. Then you are able to check whether the randomization has worked, by comparing the groups in respect of important baseline characteristics and showing that no known serious imbalance exists.

Validity

Validity refers to honesty and accuracy. If people are asked embarrassing questions or are prompted to recall events in the remote depths of their past then you may well doubt the validity of any analysis based on these data. It may be the way a particular question is worded, or the way a question sticks out like a sore thumb in a set of otherwise benign questions, or the way that you as interviewer (eg in mood, dress, attitude) have influenced the response process, or the setting in which questions are asked (eg. when other people can listen in). There may be a multitude of reasons why data may not be valid and it is up to you in your plan of action to ensure that the necessary conditions prevail to ensure validity.

There are measures which can never be valid. There is no true definition of the social world and hence no valid measure can exist of it. You shouldn't then be surprised to come across many measures of aspects of the social world being used in research, including health, intelligence, money, politics, ethnic status, housing, mental illness, environment, and occupation. Social class usually refers to a classification based on occupation and is taken to reflect the traditional social pecking order of (male) occupations.

Face validity: At the most simplistic level do the questions to be asked, or the measurements to be taken, seem sensible to you and your professional colleagues. If yes, then on the face of it or at face value you can claim to have face validity. Pilot work can clarify how sensible and unambiguous the questions are, and clearly contribute to face validity.

Content validity: Discussions with experts in the area of your research, together with an exhaustive literature and methods review should enable you to feel confident that your questions or measurements adequately cover the breadth or content of the field of study.

The setting up of a steering group to oversee the project is one way of encouraging researchers to discuss their plans more widely. Isolated researchers are less likely to be aware of the limitations of their research.

Beyond the elementary levels of face and content validity the achievement of other kinds of validity depends very much as to what is feasible and relevant.

Predictive validity: If a measurement is intended to be predictive in some way, then you have to wait and subsequently monitor what actually happens in order to assess predictive validity. For example:

Suppose it was suggested that ultrasound techniques during pregnancy were predictive of developmental outcome in early childhood.

A cohort study could be followed from early pregnancy, through birth and into early childhood.

Developmental measurements in childhood should be made by persons blind to earlier ultrasound findings.

A measurement or a question(naire) may sometimes be validated by studying distinct populations between which discrimination is expected to be at its greatest. Other groups might be chosen for which discrimination is expected to lie somewhere in-between. If the results from these different samples show the trends predicted then this is a good indicator of a valid measure:

A study assessing the validity of a questionnaire to measure pain might include a sample of subjects expected to be suffering great pain because of the nature of their condition, and another sample expected to be suffering very little pain.

Failure to discriminate between these groups on the basis of the questionnaire would argue against the validity of the questionnaire as a measure of pain.

Concurrent validity: In a sample of patients a new diagnostic test might be compared against a *reference* or established valid test. Both tests are made at the same time, ie concurrently. If a good level of agreement can be obtained then this provides evidence of validity for the new test:

---

1) Data from a self-completing questionnaire on the use of medical services could be checked against data obtained from hospital and general practitioner records.

> 2) Data from a questionnaire asking about the degree of eczema and amount of associated itching during the last month could be compared with data from a daily diary compiled by the same individuals, and with clinical assessments made at weekly intervals.

> 3) A quality of life questionnaire will embrace various aspects of living and alternative measures might be found to assess the validity of each aspect.

The validity of the reference data is obviously of crucial importance when attempting concurrent validity studies. Reference data of dubious quality is of little use for this purpose.

Reliability

Reliability refers to a method of measuring data that is consistent and repeatable.

> If you were to carry out a dental survey involving a clinical examination of children's mouths then how might you counter the criticism that there is something peculiar about the way you operate as an investigator and that this explains the results you present?
>
> You could have set aside time at the beginning of the study and asked several other dentists to repeat a series of measurements you made, and without knowledge of your findings. You could then have compared your measurements against theirs thus allowing the amount of agreement to be assessed. If there had been a lot of disagreement then the matter would have required further thought.

Such between-observer comparisons are important in the assessment of reliability. Systematic differences between observers reflect differences in judgement criteria and/or technique. If an examination or interview technique requires considerable skill and (clinical) judgement then it most likely has not been sufficiently standardised. A novice might display results which suggest a learning or training curve. Different interviewers might ask for information in different ways and thus obtain different answers.

Another way of assessing, and thereby improving, reliability is to compare one's own judgement on different occasions (within-observer reliability). For example:

> You could assess a child's mouth X-ray twice, firstly when the X-ray becomes available and secondly when all X-rays are collected together at the end of the study.
>
> For this repetition arrange for each X-ray to be devoid of any subject-identifying information so as to eliminate any conscious or sub-conscious bias on your part.

Considerable variation suggests a lack of criteria for measurement and interpretation, particularly in the hazy areas between normal and abnormal. Within-observer variation often seems random in that the direction of differences is unpredictable. Learning effects will tend to show as systematic differences.

A necessary assumption for testing within-observer reliability is that the underlying clinical state remains stable. Otherwise it is not possible to separate within-observer variation from natural patient variation:

> A repeat dental examination one year after the first is unlikely to provide suitable material for within-observer variation studies.
>
> On the other hand a self-completed questionnaire on pain repeated after a three month interval to patients with a stable chronic condition would help assess the repeatability (reliability) of the questionnaire.

Individual assessors and interviewers should be identified on study record forms. If subjects are randomly allocated to assessors then each assessor should expect in the long run to see a similar mix of subjects. A comparison of assessors in respect of subject results would then give an indication of the reliability of the assessment procedure used in the study.

A random allocation of subjects to observers is also to be encouraged for other reasons. For example:

The dental health of children attending two large schools, one private & one public is to be measured:

Dentist A has been allocated to school X.
Dentist B has been allocated to school Y.

Any comparison of schools gets confused (amongst other things) by differences in technique and judgement of the two dentists.

It would be better in the above study if each dentist carried out the same proportion of examinations in each school, and better still if children were allocated at random to the dentists.

Ideally both dentists would take part in extensive pilot work involving other dentists in order to calibrate their own techniques.

The use of a single dentist (eg dentist A only) to do all examinations from both schools would standardise the measure within the study but doesn't necessarily make the study results valid since this lone individual might be peculiar in examination habit. Pilot work involving other dentists is required to show that the lone researcher is not eccentric.

To enhance reliability and validity in any study then measurements should be made independently (blind) of the knowledge of important subgroups (eg case-control groups, randomized trial groups). This has been discussed in chapter 2. In the above example if the intention is to compare the two schools then the two dentists shouldn't be aware of which school each child attends. In practice this is difficult to achieve, and in thinking this through then time, energy, money and inconvenience have to be balanced against the greater reliability of the data. The decision will to a large extent depend on the nature of the data being collected. The number of teeth in a child's mouth should be reliably collected regardless of whether you know which school the child goes to. On the other hand a subjective assessment of the condition of the child's gums, graded as either very good, good, average, poor or very poor, may be influenced subconsciously by knowledge of the school and how this relates to the purpose of the study.

The establishment of validity and reliability is crucial for variables which relate to the main purpose of a study and every study report should make some statement on this (as should your protocol). Without such evidence the results must be viewed with caution regardless of any apparent sophistication of other aspects of design and statistical analysis. If you are using an established method which has been standardised by previous workers then the work you need to do is less than if you are trying to establish a new method of assessment. Nevertheless it cannot always be guaranteed that a method established as valid and reliable in one type of setting is automatically going to be valid and reliable in another setting.

A reliable measure may or may not be valid. For example different interviewers may all ask the same embarrassing questions in more or less the same way and obtain similar and hence reliable answers. They all may however end up with a collection of inappropriate, misleading and hence invalid answers. A machine may give similar readings regardless of who makes the reading (ie reliable in respect of operator) but if the machine is faulty then the readings are not valid. Occupational social class is a fairly reliable measure but it cannot really be considered a valid measure of the social world since it is unclear as to what the measurement is intended to reflect. An unreliable measure cannot be valid.

The pilot study phase is the time for you to iron out problems of validity and reliability, though similar work done at regular intervals in longitudinal studies is desirable to be sure of maintaining consistency in measurement. A pilot study allows you a built-in time period to take stock of any problems, to make necessary changes, and to progress with greater confidence into the major part of the investigation.

Qualitative and Quantitative methods of data collection

Qualitative methods have traditionally been regarded as yielding suspect data characterised by a loose open-ended diffuse nature. Quantitative methods on the other hand give numerical and more objective data. This, however, is too unreal and unfair a generalisation since qualitative methods can provide very valuable information. Many research projects have multiple measures of outcome and a careful choice of qualitative and quantitative methods could increase the overall information yield and hence strengthen the overall validity of the results. Thus comprehensiveness and the ability to cross-validate are enhanced. Reliability and validity are important to all methods of data collection irrespective of any nominal distinction between qualitative and quantitative methods.

Qualitative methods

Introspection. This is the observation of one's own life. One might argue that such individual data will be biased on account of one's own perception of normality and familiarity. Nevertheless such subjective data can be a useful addition to a more quantitative approach. For example a quality of life questionnaire which attempts to quantify certain aspects of health might be further enhanced by an open-ended question along the lines of:

> "At the moment, what bothers you most, if anything, about your level of health? (For example, are there things you are now unable to do as well as you used to be able to do, perhaps not at all?)"

Such qualitative methods can perhaps help the researcher understand the values and perspectives of subjects in ways often impossible when trying to summarise numerically.

Participant observation. For example a researcher becomes a tramp to study the health needs of tramps. Many aspects of an acquired lifestyle will appear strange, which reduces familiarity, but personal interpretation is a potential bias. The underlying emphasis is on observing other people by being part of their culture and recording anything of importance.

Non-participant observation. For example the observation (by video) of:

1) Behaviour patterns of mentally handicapped children.
2) Interaction between parents and children in a speech therapy program.
3) Midwife activity in a maternity unit.

There is the possibility of a Hawthorne effect, which in layman terms is no more than people behaving or reacting differently because they are aware of being observed. This can apply to all forms of data collection, numerical or otherwise, if people are conscious of their involvement in a research project.

Informal interview. This is unstructured, exploratory, and encourages people to reveal and reflect more than they might normally do. Often there is no set list of questions, merely a rough set of topics to be covered. Such sessions can be taped onto a machine for later analysis of the content of the interview. When recording informal interviews one has to be aware that the mere act of recording could affect the validity of the responses given.

Other. This includes written material such as personal diaries and letters, published commentaries, official documents and letters, minutes of meetings and policy statements of intention and direction. These tend to be shaped very much by the writer(s), and the elite do tend to be well represented. Document reviews can be conducted using a standardised format for data retrieval, with several people reviewing the same documents to assess the reliability of the method of retrieval.

Quantitative methods

Structured Interview. Questions are fixed in advance thereby allowing a uniform approach. Questions are asked in the form and in the order laid down. Answer boxes are ticked by the interviewer. The style of introduction and of any supplementary questions to clarify information already given should also be standardised to help minimise interviewer bias. Interviewers should preferably stick to questions as printed and avoid supplementary questions if possible.

To begin with it is worth piloting a range of open-ended qualitative questions in order to see the breadth of responses to each. In this way it might then be possible to close up the questions for use in a structured questionnaire with the main study sample, though a second pilot study with the improved version should also be done.

Whenever possible randomly allocate pilot subjects to several interviewers. In this way the experience of each interviewer can afterwards be discussed, as can any apparent differences between interviewers in the results obtained. Any ambiguities should be ironed out at this early stage in the proceedings.

Interview questionnaires totally comprised of precoded answers are generally unsatisfactory to both the respondent and the interviewer, and ultimately to the researcher. Some people may feel frustrated at being constrained at the choice of answer on offer and at being unable to express their answer in their own terms. The interview might then take on an air of artificiality with the interviewer perhaps assuming an authoritarian role and thereby perhaps producing artificial answers. It is therefore useful to include some open-ended questions even if they cannot be analysed numerically by statistical methods. They will add to the comprehensiveness and enhance the overall validity of results.

Self-completing questionnaire. Subjects are handed or posted a questionnaire to complete and return. Most questions offer a range of precoded answers though it is useful, as for interview questionnaires, to have some open-ended questions to allow respondents the opportunity of expressing any feelings inadequately covered by the questionnaire.

A lot of preparation work should go into the layout, instructions, and the wording of questions, to ensure that the respondent is aware of what is required. In the main study there may be no one around who can be asked to clarify any ambiguity, and so the questionnaire should be extensively piloted beforehand.

Initially it is worthwhile devising open-ended questions to see the range of answers that people give. It is then easier to decide how to pre-code the answers in the final version. Your first attempts at pre-coding need to be cross-checked for problems of ambiguity. Each pilot subject can be handed a questionnaire and asked to complete it, whilst you are on hand to answer any problems the respondent has with its completion. You can then go through the answers of each question in turn with the respondent in order to try and understand the meaning that he/she has attached to each question. Find several other people who will administer the pilot questionnaire in this way. Then you can all meet up to discuss experiences and to refine the questionnaire further.

Questionnaire design can be very time-consuming and requires pilot work. Some off-the-shelf questionnaires have been tested out (for reliability and validity) under varying circumstances and it is always worth seeing if any of these are suitable for your purpose. And, no matter how good the recommendation, please pilot it out in your own situation since there is no automatic guarantee that questionnaires travel well.

Clinical measurements and laboratory values. Data are recorded as numbers or pre-coded categories and are stored for the purpose of research onto a record form. Sections for open-ended comment may also be included, eg to describe the use of prescribed drug therapies. Requirements for establishing reliability and validity apply as much to these types of measurement as to any other.

Sometimes a choice between a self-completion questionnaire and an interview questionnaire has to be made. It is possible that the two methods could give different answers. The self-completion questionnaire tends to be cheaper and allows a greater number of subjects to be studied. It also allows respondents to complete their answers at their own speed. It is also more likely to be reliable. Potential disadvantages are poor comprehension, questions may be left unanswered, there is no supplementary probing and response by post may be poor. With interviewing the interviewers have to be trained and paid, and there may be considerable interviewer bias. A smaller number of respondents is likely to be enrolled for study, though the information on each is more likely to be complete and there is more scope for asking in-depth questions. The ultimate choice should ideally be made with the purpose of the research clearly in mind.

Both self-completion and interview methods can be used in the same study. In this way an interview can tackle issues in some depth in a few (as representative as possible) subjects. Meanwhile a self-completion questionnaire can provide a more general set of responses from a much larger number of people. The results from the interview could be used to complement the more superficial but numerical data from the questionnaire.

A study may thus involve a mixture of data collection methods:

An audit of an alcohol detoxification unit could include: Statements of unit policy and intent, minutes of meetings, priorities for treatment and criteria for appropriate treatment, descriptive surveys of the case-mix seen, longitudinal studies of patients through the unit to predict which patients seem to do best and which do worst and to identify inappropriate practices, questionnaire surveys of patient (& family) expectations from treatment and of satisfaction from the services on offer, interviews with staff members about job satisfaction and treatment priorities and preferences, non-participant observation of interaction between staff and patients, questionnaire surveys of GP's and hospital consultants who refer patients to the unit as to what kind of service they would like. Followed by Action and Re-Audit.

Quality of life

The concept of quality of life is perhaps better described in medical research as health status, taking into account the feelings and subjective physical and social well-being of the patient. The ideal is for well defined instruments that can be applied and interpreted easily and for which there is no great burden of labour.

There has to be compromise between the pragmatic yearnings for an easily administered tailor-made instrument with questions specifically addressing the study's immediate concerns (eg pain) and the wider scientific demands of comprehensiveness (ie areas other than pain), validity and reliability. You may feel the need to develop your own questions, though first you should perhaps consider the full range of off the shelf instruments already available. Your own questions (eg on pain) may seem more directly applicable but do require development to be convincing and often this important aspect is ignored. The compromise would be to choose a more general off the shelf instrument together with specific questions devised in addition if these highlight key symptoms or side-effects associated with the condition or treatment of patients.

In clinical studies a most useful category of health status measurement is a measure of perceived health. A patient-derived measure of health status should be regarded as one of the longer term outcomes. Whereas biochemical or physiological changes tend to be more rapid, health measures reflecting social and emotional change may require a much longer time to come into effect. You should think about using health status measures over periods of months and years rather than days and weeks. It is for this reason that such measures are not particularly suited for the cross-over type of study. If patients are quite ill then the relative simplicity of a measure could make it an attractive choice especially if several repeated observations are to be made over time.

Health status measures are suitable for cost-benefit analyses, in randomized clinical evaluations, and in population-based studies. The multi-dimensionality of a health status measure has often been raised in argument against its use in that you would need to trade off results from one dimension against another. This hints at the desirability of a single global index, or score, embracing all possible dimensions. The problem in this, as with the combination of any outcome measures that are different, is the loss of sensitivity to subtle and perhaps important changes. There is no single clinical, physiological or biochemical measure of health and no logical reason for imagining that any single value could possibly summarise perceived health. It would seem to make more sense for you to discuss improvements in specific areas rather than in terms of any overall score.

The wording of questions

Research is all about asking questions. These appear in interviews, self-completing questionnaires and in record sheets designed to capture clinical examinations, assessments and laboratory measurements. Deciding which is the best question to use and how best to set it out on paper is often a matter of common-sense and it is difficult here to generalise to all situations. This section offers you an overview and makes a number of suggestions. For simplicity let us refer to self-completed questionnaires, interview questionnaires, and clinical assessment sheets collectively as record forms, that is as sheets or forms that act as a study record for the collected data.

If a few highly trained individuals are collecting data from subjects then they can usually be relied upon to turn to and follow quite detailed instructions. If the record form is to be filled in by a large number of semi-trained and generally less motivated people then instructions need to be simple and clear. Members of the public cannot be relied upon to read and remember extensive footnotes for example. Every question should be self-explanatory.

Put general instructions for filling in a record form at the top of the form. On self-completing questionnaires some indication of the reason for doing the study is helpful since a natural reaction to any form is "why should I bother to fill this in?". An alternative would be to carefully word an accompanying letter.

If you want to sample from the lists of a general practice then an accompanying letter signed and supported by each member of the practice can help to emphasise the importance of the research, re-assure the subject, and help boost the response rate.

There may sometimes be, depending on the nature of the study, a fine dividing line between persuasion and perceived coercion. This is discussed in chapter 3 as informed consent. Subjects may try to please you with their answers so as to preserve their doctor-patient relationship.

Put specific instructions and clarifications for particular questions alongside each question. The drafting of clear unambiguous questions is time consuming. Some people find the completion of any form a difficult task. This difficulty could manifest itself through non-response.

Slight subtle variations of wording can make a big difference to the answers you get. Define the issues of interest and word questions very carefully. Only have one idea per question. Use simple words that won't confuse people.

The yes/no is the easiest type of closed question to handle though information may sometimes be lost by the failure to discriminate in any greater depth. Categories like severe/moderate/mild/none may sometimes be appropriate.

Define alternative responses carefully and be wary of an imbalance in alternatives offered:

> 1) Extremely satisfied,
> 2) Fairly satisfied,
> 3) Not satisfied
>
> is unbalanced whereas:
>
> 1) Very satisfied,
> 2) Satisfied,
> 3) Dis-satisfied,
> 4) Very dissatisfied
>
> is weighted equally positively & negatively.

There is a natural tendency for people to respond to a middle or soft option should one be offered. Trying to force an opinion by the use of "yes" and "no" as answers to some controversial question may give a different distribution of responses than if the option "don't know" is offered as well. The middle option can be used if the wish is to draw out strong convictions one way or another. Those who feel reluctant to answer "yes" or "no" can then with safety answer "don't know". The middle option can be left out if the wish is to measure tendencies or leanings. Thus those offered "yes" and "no" as the only alternatives are forced to choose one or other even if they feel little leaning one way or another. Some people may actually write or verbally offer "don't know" as an alternative.

A 4 point scale (eg very happy, happy, unhappy, very unhappy) is a good compromise, allowing some discrimination between strongly held and less extreme feelings. Such a scale might be combined with the giving of statements. Thus a subject may be asked to read a number of statements and to indicate their level of agreement with each statement:

```
The NHS provides value for money:

        1) Strongly agree,
        2) Agree,
        3) Disagree,
        4) Strongly disagree.
```

A 5 point scale allows a middle option as well (eg strongly agree, agree, undecided, disagree, strongly disagree).

An analogue scale may also have its uses. For example subjects are asked to describe the degree of pain they are suffering and they are shown a horizontal scale ranging from no pain at one end to excruciating pain at the other end. They are then asked to make a mark along this horizontal scale to indicate their level of pain. The distance from the no pain end of the scale to the mark can then be measured by a ruler:

```
"Make a mark along this horizontal scale to indicate the level of pain you are
suffering":-

        no pain]-------X-------------------------------[excruciating pain
                       mark
```

Every question should require an answer from the person completing the record form:

```
        Does your child wet the bed?
```

A "yes" response is a clear positive response but no answer at all (ie left "blank") or a dash ("-") is by no means a clear negative response. It may mean "no" though other meanings are possible. "Inapplicable" (ie no child), "don't know", "refused to answer", "forgot to answer" (ie I'll answer that one later) are all variations which might need to be distinguished and given separate boxes and codes:

Does your child wet the bed? (Tick one box only)		
	1. Yes	[ ]
	2. No	[ ]
	3. Don't know	[ ]
	4. No Children	[ ]

The open-ended form of question is hard to code, but if the answers need to be coded (eg for computer analysis) then this coding can only be done with effect after the data have been collected and the range of answers scanned through. Thus *How do you feel about the way you were looked after in hospital?* is an open-ended question and the answers may be wide ranging. Only on seeing this range can some numerical codes be assigned to the different kinds of answers given. Favourable answers might be coded as 1, unfavourable as 2. Several people should assess the answers and produce their own codings, as a check on the reliability of the coding procedure.

Do try out subtle variations in the wording of questions and in the closed options you offer as answers, to see if such changes do have any pronounced effect on the answers given. You may be surprised in your pilot work as to how important this is.

Pilot study work is a very important part of questionnaire design and shouldn't be under-estimated nor skated over.

Layout of record forms and the computer handling of data

Unless you analyse your data by hand (recommended if you have a very small number of questions and no detailed analyses planned) you will no doubt be looking to use a computer for the input of data and for the analysis. If you hope to make use of a computer department or bureau then it would be to your advantage to discuss your plans for data capture with them before you embark on the study. Time-consuming problems could arise involving you in needless transcription of data and it is better spending time to sort out the layout of record forms at the outset. Try and avoid the transcription process by designing record forms that serve both the needs of manual and computer systems.

Computer operators are the people who punch in data from computer keyboards to computer disks. They like to see a record form with numbers presented to them in a clear logical order. A good record form layout reduces the chance of error when data is typed into a computer system. My personal preference in the layout of record forms is for a right hand margin space in which computer boxes can be placed. You or the computer operator need then only scan down this right hand margin in order to enter the data.

The fictitious example on the next page illustrates how different types of questions can be organised onto the same record form. A layout of this type suitable for computer processing can be achieved for both interview and self-completing questionnaires as well as for the recording of clinical assessments.

The left side and main part of the form acts as the manual record. Transcription of appropriate numbers into the right side computer margin enables easy computer processing. For example if the child is a girl then the value of 2 is placed in the box in the computer margin. The blood test results can be placed directly on the form margin so as to reduce transcription workload. Answers to open-ended questions can be coded numerically and a box has been allocated in the computer margin just in case one is needed.

Each record form should have its own unique computer serial number. This can be the subject's study number. Then any errors in the computer data can easily be traced back to the record form. It also avoids the need to input names and addresses, thereby helping to protect computer held data from abuse.

The desired accuracy of a clinical measurement can be specified by the insertion of the required number of boxes onto the record form. For example [ ][ ].[ ] would imply that accuracy to one decimal place was required whilst [ ][ ].[ ][ ] would imply two decimal places. This avoids the common problem of different assessors recording data to their own chosen level of accuracy.

The use of the codes 9, 99, 999, 99.9 etc are often reserved for the "don't know" or "missing" categories and values, assuming that these are out of the range of possible real values.

Example to illustrate record form layout

Name of child_____   [ ][ ][ ] serial number

Age of child last birthday ? _____years   [ ][ ] years

Sex of child   [ ] 1.boy
               [ ] 2.girl   [ ] sex

How would you describe your child's health at present?

         [ ] 1.very good
         [ ] 2.good
         [ ] 3.fair
         [ ] 4.poor
         [ ] 5.very poor   [ ]

At the moment what bothers you most, if anything, about your child's level of health ?

....
....
....   [ ]

Clinical diagnosis   [ ] 1.chronic liver disease
                 [ ] 2.malignancy
                 [ ] 3.other   [ ]

Give details:

....
....   [ ]
....

Blood Results:

Haemoglobin	[ ][ ].[ ]
Creatinine	[ ][ ][ ][ ]
Urea	[ ][ ].[ ]
Potassium	[ ][ ].[ ]
Albumin	[ ][ ][ ]

If you have never punched data into a computer system then it is a useful experience to put yourself through since you will gain a much better feel for the variations within a dataset.

Further reading (See Chapter 9 for full list of references):

Ref 1 (chpt 4)
Ref 2 (chpt 27)
Ref 5 (chpt 11)
Ref 6 (p18-21, p26-30)
Ref's 11, 13, 32, 41

6. DATA SUMMARY

By reading through this chapter you will build upon your literature & methods review and better understand the ways in which you can summarise, or describe, your results. Imagine yourself at a conference and about to present your main overhead transparencies in a five minute time slot. What tables and pictures would you want to show? This may now seem light years ahead to you, yet to think in this way will make you much more aware of the data you need to collect, and of the numbers of subjects that are needed.

Draft out these tables and pictures now if you can, and revise them later after reading this chapter. Make an educated guess at the numbers of subjects in any subgroups you have identified, paying special regard to the method of recruiting subjects. It may be that you need to over-sample in one subgroup in order to produce enough subjects in another subgroup. From this rather simplistic but realistic exercise obtain your first estimate of sample size. This will be refined later.

Description and inference

Description and summary, through tables, summary statistics and pictures is an important first stage of analysis. This chapter suggests various ways to describe and summarise data, including some that might be new to you.

Inference from the sample to the wider population through probability based methods is the next stage. The use of confidence intervals and tests of significance, assumes a probability model for the data. One part of this inferential phase of analysis is looking for simple methods, possibly graphical, by which any conclusions can be easily presented.

When you first begin your write up of results, begin with a report of the results without any mention of tests of statistical significance or of confidence intervals. So much can be gained by simply looking at your data and by not rushing hell for leather into tests of statistical significance. A simple rule of thumb for you is to plan to spend more time in just looking at your data. You will then gain a better feeling for what it is saying to you. Let the trends in the data emerge, and make a note of any interesting observations. Then, and only then, compute the relevant confidence intervals or tests of significance, ie those that relate to the hypotheses and expectations declared before your study began. The methods of statistical inference thus become an added refinement to an analysis that is primarily descriptive.

The next chapter considers statistical inference in more detail, and gets under the surface to see how sample sizes can be better estimated. The rest of this chapter concentrates on methods of description with an emphasis on the appropriateness of each rather than on "how to do". There are ample references at the end of the chapter to allow you to dig deeper into any area that you feel is important to you. The intention is to point you in the right direction, to give you reasoned choice, but if you do feel out of your depth then please do point yourself towards your friendly statistician.

In your protocol say how you will analyse your data.

Checking data

The first computer programs you run should check for coding and punching errors. Look out for values that are logically inconsistent and in conflict with expected ranges or possibilities. A third or fourth code for gender would suggest an error either in transcription or in punching. A birthweight of 3500 grams and a gestation of 24 weeks would have to be cross-checked.

To do this in a systematic way scan down the frequency distribution for each variable and work out a list of two-variable and multi-variable consistency cross-checks. Incorporate these checks into a computer program that will flag any inconsistencies. Some systems allow checks to form part of data entry and data won't be accepted into the database unless the specified conditions are satisfied. Check all extremes (outliers) in your dataset but always retain them unless there is very clear evidence for excluding them.

Ironing out errors is always time well spent and it is much better to do this early on. Otherwise errors are later unearthed one by one and the programs have to be re-run again and again.

Variables

It is useful to distinguish different types of variable because different methods of analysis apply. The prime division is into Qualitative and Quantitative variables:

Qualitative: or categorical, non-numerical:

eg. type of drug (A,B,C)
  outcome (alive,dead)
  severity of pain (none,mild,moderate,severe)

Categorical variables either have some underlying natural order (ordinal) or have no natural ordering (nominal). A common type with only two categories is also called binary.

Quantitative: numerical, count or measurement.

  a) discrete:
  eg. number of aneurysms
  number of children in family
  number of teeth missing
  b) continuous:
  eg. Height,weight,blood pressure,serum
  cholesterol

Tables and figures

Tables are used extensively to present data. You should distinguish between tables for reference where the worth of the table lies with the tabulated values for future reference, and tables for demonstration which are to make a point. For demonstration tables the numbers can be simplified, rounded to a few significant figures. It is for demonstration purposes that pictures or figures may be preferable to tables. The difficulty of preparation has to be balanced against the ability to convey the desired message. There are a wide variety of ways of presenting data pictorially. Remember the Chinese proverb "a picture tells a thousand words".

Avoid making tables and figures unnecessarily complex and so cluttered up with detail that their impact and message is reduced. They should always have a title and be self-explanatory. It is frustrating to the reader to have to search around within the text of a report for clues as to the meaning of tables.

Frequencies and Frequency Distributions

<u>Qualitative</u>

The following example introduces the terms *frequency* and *relative frequency* and indicates the commonly used ways of displaying qualitative data:

> Of 200 people 120 are male and 80 are female. The counts 120 and 80 are known as frequencies, the total count of 200 being the total frequency. Thus 60% of the sample are male and 40% female, the 60% and 40% being the relative frequencies of males and females.

Frequency and relative frequency distributions of qualitative data are often shown in Bar-charts and Pie-Charts. Bar-charts can be displayed horizontally or vertically with the length of the bar representing the frequency, or relative frequency as appropriate (see Figure 6.1). Pie-charts (not shown) are drawn as circles, divided up so that the areas of the segments represent the frequencies.

As you can see from Figure 6.1 the Bar-chart allows a particularly good visual comparison of two or more groups to be made.

Figure 6.1 Drug therapy and outcome in a randomized clinical trial

Clinical Outcome	Drug Therapy		
	Drug 1	Drug 2	Drug 3
Fully Employable	108	152	112
Alive but not fully employable	58	28	41
Dead 1 - 3 months after treatment	39	40	41
Dead within 28 days of treatment	35	12	54

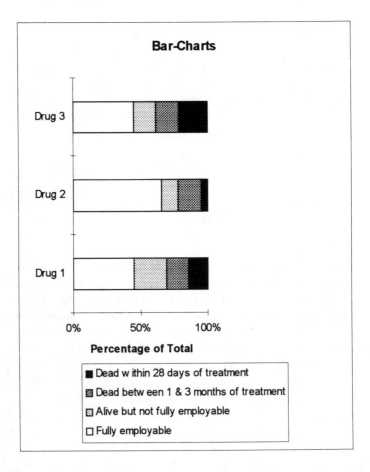

Quantitative

A useful first step is to arrange the data in ascending order and form a frequency distribution. A stem and leaf plot can be a good way of beginning this. For example the following data:

10.2	11.4	12.4	11.4	10.3	10.9	10.6	10.8
11.5	12.6	11.8	10.8	10.8	10.5	10.1	11.2
10.5	10.6	11.3	11.2	10.7	10.9	11.1	11.0
12.1	10.0	12.2	11.8	10.8	10.6	10.9	11.1
12.9	10.6	10.5	11.1	10.9	10.8	10.8	10.7

can be shown thus:

stem	leaf
10	01235556666778888889999
11	011122344588
12	12469

The frequency distribution could also be shown in the form of a simple dot plot:

```
                          .
                          .
                      .  ..
                     ..  ..  .
                     ..... ..  .      .
                 ....  ...........   .  ..  .    .
                 ------------------------------
      leaf       01234567890123456789 0123456789
      stem       10          11          12
```

Another easy way of displaying a frequency or relative frequency distribution is by drawing a frequency polygon (see Table 6.1 and Figure 6.2). This is achieved by computing grouped frequencies and by joining up the midpoints of the relevant groups. At either end the frequency polygon line is joined to the horizontal axis (ie zero frequency) at the midpoints of the groups just above and below. One advantage of using the frequency polygon (rather than the commonly used histogram) is the ability to convey several frequency distributions within the same picture frame, for example the weights of males and females.

Most quantitative frequency distributions encountered in medicine have only one peak. Most tend to be either symmetrical or skewed off to the right. Typically, we think of a symmetrical distribution shaped like a bell and tailing off in both directions. A skew to the right is *positive* and a skew to the left is *negative*. Note that the distribution of weights in Figure 6.2 is skewed slightly to the right. A distribution of the period of gestation in a sample of pregnant women shows a skew to the left.

Another good way of displaying a frequency distribution, and one which avoids the grouping of values into intervals is the cumulative frequency plot. The horizontal axis of the plot represents the scale of measurement of the variable (eg weight). The vertical axis can be scaled according to the cumulative frequency as in Figure 6.2. [It can also be scaled from zero to 100 percent thereby giving the cumulative relative frequency plot.] For any value on the horizontal axis, it is possible to read off from the vertical axis the percentage of sample observations at or below that value. In Figure 6.2 the percentage of males weighing 76 Kg or under is about 50%. The cumulative plot can also compare two or more distributions on the same picture.

Table 6.1 Weights in Kg (to nearest Kg) of 130 men

```
66 77 71 83 75 85 72 81 64 65 76 81 86 73 79 72 77 68 72 70
79 71 79 77 77 77 79 86 90 76 84 75 79 95 81 83 85 82 71
89 79 76 70 78 79 77 70 84 74 68 80 66 78 72 92 66 95 67 79
67 72 75 72 73 72 74 78 75 81 70 86 67 77 68 80 74 86 64 81
67 73 73 78 66 66 70 74 73 67 83 79 67 69 73 75 77 79 72 80
88 86 85 81 67 78 73 69 72 76 67 89 94 67 67 75 87 65 99 75
76 66 97 86 88 80 77 76 79 69
```

weight	frequency	cumulative frequency	weight	frequency	cumulative frequency
64	2	2	80	4	96
65	2	4	81	6	102
66	6	10	82	1	103
67	10	20	83	3	106
68	3	23	84	2	108
69	3	26	85	3	111
70	5	31	86	6	117
71	3	34	87	1	118
72	9	43	88	2	120
73	7	50	89	2	122
74	4	54	90	1	123
75	7	61	92	1	124
76	6	67	94	1	125
77	9	76	95	3	128
78	5	81	97	1	129
79	11	92	99	1	130

Table 6.1 (Continued)				
Weight Group	Group Frequency		Weight Group	Group Frequency
60-4	2		80-4	16
65-9	24		85-9	14
70-4	28		90-4	3
75-9	38		95-9	5

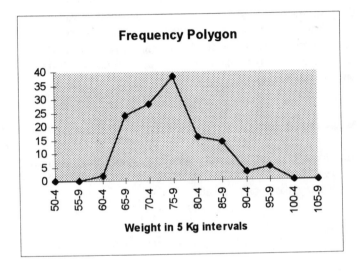

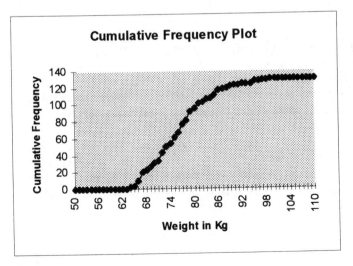

Summary Statistics

It is often desirable and convenient to express key aspects of a frequency distribution by one or two summary statistics. Sometimes a single percentage may suffice such as the percentage of mothers with more than 2 children, the percentage of patients with hypertension, the percentage with severe pain, the percentage with type A blood. For a quantitative variable the key aspects are usually a measure of the centre of the distribution (eg mean, median) and a measure of the scatter or variability of the distribution (eg standard deviation, interquartile range).

Mean and Median

The **mean** of a set of measurements is simply their numerical average obtained by adding them all up and dividing by the number of measurements. Thus:

Mean of (18,20,22,23,24,24,25,26,28,30) is 24

This mean of 24 is a value representative of the centre of the distribution of measurements. However:

Mean of (18,20,22,23,24,24,25,26,52,96) is 33

This mean of 33 is not typical of the centre of the set of values. In general the mean fails to represent the centre of a distribution when the shape of that distribution is markedly skewed.

The mean should only really be used for data measured on what is called an interval scale, when one can attach the same meaning to equally spaced intervals anywhere along the scale (such as for height or weight):

Consider a subjective scoring scale, moving from 1=very satisfied to 4=very dissatisfied.

Suppose that the jump from 1=very satisfied to 2=satisfied on this scale represents a considerably smaller degree of change than from 2=satisfied to 3=disatisfied.

To report in a longitudinal study that the mean change in satisfaction of males was from 1.5 to 2.3 units and in females from 2.4 to 3.2 units would imply an average change of 0.8 for both sexes.

It would be misleading to say there was little difference on average in the way male and female satisfaction changed over time, since the females clearly experienced a more important degree of change.

Scoring systems like these are commonly used but are potentially confusing. You are better off reporting percentages (of v satisfied, satisfied, dissatisfied, v dissatisfied).

The **median** is the value that splits a distribution of values exactly in half. If all values were ordered from lowest to highest then the median would be the middle value. Thus:

Median of (18,20,22,23,24,24,25,26,28,30) is 24

The above median is the simple average of the fifth and sixth observations. If there had been eleven rather than ten observations then the median would have been equal to the sixth observation in the ordered list.

Median of (18,20,22,23,24,24,25,26,52,96) is 24

Thus the median has the advantage of being insensitive to outlying values.

The median is generally a better descriptive measure of the centre of a frequency distribution than the mean. When the distribution is symmetrical then the two should more or less agree.

The mean's nicer mathematical properties however makes it more suited for the methods of statistical inference. This explains the desire for distributions with one peak that display symmetry. It also explains why you might use transformation techniques (eg taking logarithmic values) to try and bring about symmetry in the transformed scale when the original scale is skewed. The mean of the appropriately transformed data can then be taken as the statistic describing the centre of the distribution of values.

Quantiles

The median can also be called the 50th percentile of the distribution. It is the value at or below which fifty percent of the frequencies lie. It can be read off from a cumulative (relative) frequency plot (see Figure 6.2) as can any other percentile points (or quantiles), such as the 25th and 75th quantiles.

The most direct way of summarising a frequency distribution is to give a set of quantile values. This is particularly relevant for the establishment of a reference (or often termed "normal") range of values. Often it seems to be that some quantile out in the tail of the distribution is of greatest interest, such as the 95th percentile above which only five percent of the sample values lies.

Mode

The mode measures the peak in a frequency distribution. It is difficult to use in a small sample of continuous data and is of little relevance in a large sample. The mode can more meaningfully be given for categorical data when it simply becomes that category which appears most frequently.

Range, Interquartile Range and Standard Deviation

The range of a distribution is from the lowest value to the highest value. By itself the range is of limited use since it is sensitive to extreme outlying values. It also depends on the sample size in that the more subjects you have the wider apart the extreme values are likely to be.

Scatter can better be summarised by quoting quantile ranges such as the gap between the 10th and 90th percentiles or between the 25th and 75th. The gap between the 25th and 75th percentiles is called the interquartile range and gives the two values between which the middle half of the distribution of ordered values lie. Thus 25 percent of values will lie at or below the 25th percentile value and 25 percent will lie above the 75th percentile, leaving 50 percent in-between.

Together the median and interquartile range can summarise the centre and the spread of a distribution of values. You can also quote the upper and lower values of the range as these will point to any extreme values in the distribution. A graphical representation of all this is provided by a Box and Whisker Plot (see Figure 6.3). The box part of the plot is formed by drawing a rectangle, defined by the 75th and 25th percentile values. The box is divided into two by the median value. Extending from the box are two straight lines resembling whiskers which represent the lower and upper reaches of the distribution. Should there be any very extreme values then the length of the whiskers can be set to one and a half times the length of the box and individual points outside this can be plotted separately. The box and whisker plot is a good way to visually assess symmetry of a frequency distribution and indeed it provides a clear simple picture of the distribution as a whole. Several distributions can be contrasted side by side.

Figure 6.3: Box and whisker plots

DATASET A	DATASET B
170 165 185 174 179 177 166 181	20 111 110 31 591 577 84 340
175 184 164 177 186 180 178 187	396 32 155 74 186 160 15 599
172 182 181 172 185 186 176 183	470 30 450 253 138 153 94 118
170 180 186 178 181 177 179 183	76 18 765 393 59 238 42 140
173 186 176 180 185 181 187 175	148 22 665 615 23 357 491 10
172 160 177 166 182 171 185 188	102 4 178 137 93 719 338 39
179 167 176 174 162 178 172 181	423 264 112 116 49 136 292 17
177 188 170 157 176 163 177 189	325 345 69 249 17 150 154 78
179 182 167 171 183 178 196 172	42 293 49 344 936 27 157 67
164 176 183 177 189 175 173 197	158 33 12 248 52 71 432 252
178 169 193 177 182 168 192 190	188 154 30 238 889 28 404 316
183 171 168 194 171 168 173 193	15 212 23 30 110 40 244 257
179 191 166 178	49 206 212 29

FREQUENCY DISTRIBUTIONS

Interval	Frequency		Interval	Frequency
155-9	1		0-19	8
160-4	5		20-39	14
165-9	10		40-59	8
170-4	17		60-79	6
175-9	27		80-99	3
180-4	18		100-49	12
185-9	14		150-99	11
190-4	6		200-49	8
195-9	2		250-99	6
			300-99	9
			400-599	9
			600-799	4
			800-999	2

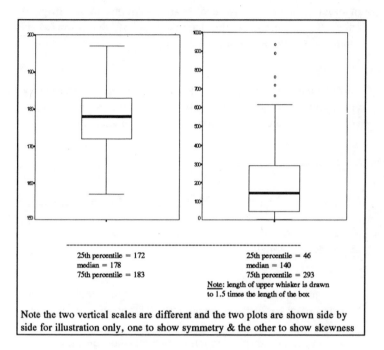

```
25th percentile = 172                    25th percentile = 46
median = 178                             median = 140
75th percentile = 183                    75th percentile = 293
                              Note: length of upper whisker is drawn
                                   to 1.5 times the length of the box
```

Note the two vertical scales are different and the two plots are shown side by side for illustration only, one to show symmetry & the other to show skewness

The interquartile range is a good descriptive statistic for scatter. However it doesn't lend itself easily towards methods of statistical inference. A measure of scatter with good mathematical properties is the variance, and derived from this it's square root the standard deviation.

The variance is the average of the squared deviations from the mean value and it's computation is as follows:

The mean is subtracted from each of the measurements in turn. These differences, some negative some positive, are the deviations from the mean. Convention is to square each of the deviations and then to add all these squared deviations together. The variance is then equal to this sum of squared deviations divided by one less than the number of measurements in the set of data.

In order to have a measure of scatter in terms of the original units of measurement the square root of the variance is computed to give the **standard deviation**.

The variance and standard deviation will increase as the scatter of measurements about the mean value increases and they are very sensitive to extreme outlying values. For example:

Variance of (18,20,22,23,24,24,25,26,28,30) is 13

Variance of (18,20,22,23,24,24,25,26,52,96) is 580

Bell-shaped symmetry

The frequency distribution that a mean and standard deviation best describes has bell-like symmetry. The mean plus or minus one standard deviation will include about two-thirds of all values and the mean plus or minus two standard deviations will include about 95 percent of all values. These rules of thumb are based on a theoretical distribution called the normal distribution. For example:

The frequency distribution of 500 male heights shows a bell-like symmetry. The mean height is 175cms and the standard deviation is 8cms. From this you can say that about two-thirds of the heights are between 167 and 183 cms and about 95% are between 159 and 191 cms.

You can say a lot of other things too from the mean and standard deviation, about the frequency distribution, so long as the distribution shows this bell-like symmetry.

If the shape of a frequency distribution is highly skewed then the mean gives a poor description of the centre of the distribution whilst the standard deviation becomes enormous. For example:

In a study of water transit times a sample mean of 1.24 seconds and standard deviation of 5.56 seconds are reported. Both the mean and standard deviation are inappropriate summary statistics for this distribution of water transit times, as we shall now see.

Imagine a bell-like distribution with mean 1.24 seconds and standard deviation 5.56 seconds. This is what these statistics describe. Mean ± One standard deviation gives the range from -4.32 seconds to 6.80 seconds.

Thus about two-thirds of water transit times are between -4.32 seconds and 6.80 seconds. This is clearly nonsense since negative times are impossible. Yet to follow logically what the mean and standard deviation are saying, you are being asked to believe that nearly half the water transit times are negative.

All that can be said about the frequency distribution of this variable is that the centre of the distribution is some way below the value of 1.24 and that there is a large skew to the right with a few very long water transit times.

In the above example it would be better to either seek some form of data transformation so that the frequency distribution of the transformed variable shows bell-like symmetry and can be summarised by a mean and standard deviation, or to summarise the frequency distribution using quantiles.

You may already have plans for means and standard deviations to be worked out for you by computer, and the computer will dutifully cough up the numbers. But don't forget to ask it for the pictures as well! Spend more time looking at the shape of frequency distributions before you give a condensed summary of them.

Attributable Risk, Relative Risk, & Odds Ratio

Attributable risks and Relative risks are summary statistics derived directly from incidence, and are used to report longitudinal studies:

Attributable risk measures the arithmetic difference between incidences (of disease) in exposed and unexposed groups.

Relative risk measures the ratio of incidences in exposed and unexposed groups.

An example has already been given in chapter two, within the section describing incidence and prevalence studies.

The odds ratio is a statistic often used in case-control studies to provide an estimate of relative risk and it gives a good approximation if the disease in question is rare. For example:

		CASES (disease)	CONTROLS (no disease)
CHARACTERISTIC OF INTEREST (exposure)	male	115	40
	female	185	260
	total	300	300

For cases the odds in favour of males are 115 to 185.

For controls the odds in favour of males are 40 to 260.

The odds ratio is thus 115/185 divided by 40/260 = 4.04

Measures of Association

An association or correlation between two categorical variables can easily be shown by bar-charts, as for example in Figure 6.1. The distribution of clinical outcome for patients in each of three drug groups can be easily compared. Visually the bars look different, with those patients receiving drug 2 doing better than patients receiving drugs 1 & 3. In other words there seems to be an association between drug use and clinical outcome.

An association between a binary and a quantitative variable can be shown by a dot-plot. For example:

```
Haemoglobin levels:
                        .
                      ...
Drug                  ....
Group               ........
(n=47)            ............
          .  ................. .
          -----------------------------------
leaf      0123456789012345678901234567890123
stem      10        11        12        13      Hb
leaf      0123456789012345678901234567890123
          -----------------------------------
                              ..............
Placebo                    .  ...........
Group                         ........
(n=42)                         .....
                                ...
                                 .
```

Frequency polygons, cumulative (relative) frequency plots, and box & whisker plots are also ways of comparing two distributions. They can be used to compare three or more distributions.

An association between two quantitative variables is easily shown in a scatter plot showing all pairs of values (Figure 6.4):

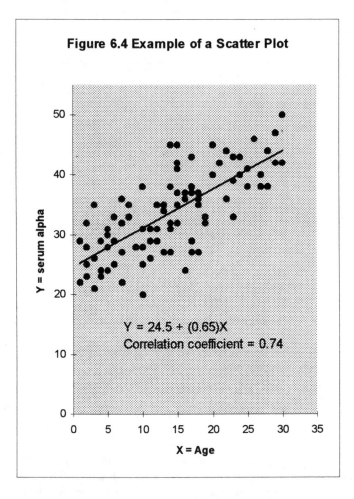

Figure 6.4 Example of a Scatter Plot

Y = 24.5 + (0.65)X
Correlation coefficient = 0.74

Y = serum alpha

X = Age

Regression and Correlation

To make this section easier to digest think of X as age in years and of Y as some biochemical measurement.

Least squares linear regression techniques will give you the equation of the best fitting straight-line relationship between two variables. A scatter plot shows whether this straight-line does indeed describe the relationship between Y and X (as in Figure 6.4). If the relationship between Y and X is curved, or if one or both frequency distributions are severely skewed, then the straight-line equation by itself as a summary will mislead. Transformations of one or both variables may help. Always check that the computed equation can be seen to fit the data.

The (Pearson) correlation coefficient measures how closely the data points are scattered about a regression line. A lot of scatter suggests a correlation coefficient close to zero whilst very little scatter suggests a coefficient close to $+1$ or -1. The equation $Y = 24.5 + 0.65X$ (see Figure 6.4) implies a positive relationship in that as X increases then Y increases and the correlation coefficient of 0.74 measures the strength of the positive relationship.

A very useful statistic describing the closeness of scatter of points about a regression line is the square of the correlation coefficient. This can be interpreted as the proportion of variance in Y that can be explained away by knowing X. It is the variability in Y that we seek to explain away or predict. Squaring a correlation coefficient of 0.74 gives a value of 0.55 and this means that 55% of all the scatter in Y values can be accounted for by a linear relationship between X and Y. Most importantly here perhaps is the information that almost one-half of the variation in Y values has not been accounted for.

Always look at the scatterplot before placing your trust in correlation coefficients and regression equations. A computer can easily churn out the numbers. Get it to draw the plots as well.

Multiple regression

You would consider this approach when there are several continuous predictor or explanatory variables (eg X1, X2, X3) and a single continuous dependent variable (eg Y). For example:

X1 (age in years)
X2 (weight in Kg)
X3 (height in cms)
Y (Blood serum alpha Y)

An equation:

BLOOD SERUM $Y = 1000 + (2.4)AGE + (0.4)WEIGHT - (1.5)HEIGHT$

allows the prediction of BLOOD SERUM Y for different values of AGE, WEIGHT & HEIGHT. It is assumed that AGE, WEIGHT, & HEIGHT each separately have a linear predictive effect on BLOOD SERUM Y, because it is this relationship with Y that has been entered into the model to produce the above best fitting equation. However the equation fails to indicate the relative importance of AGE, WEIGHT and HEIGHT nor does it indicate how much variation in BLOOD SERUM Y can be accounted for by these three variables. There is a statistic, the square of the multiple correlation coefficient, that can give such information, as in this example:

	PREDICTOR VARIABLES	VARIATION IN Y ACCOUNTED FOR
age	X1 only	36%
weight	X2 only	8%
height	X3 only	15%
age & weight	X1 and X2	37%
age & height	X1 and X3	49%
weight & height	X2 and X3	17%
age, weight & height	X1 and X2 and X3	50%

Thus AGE alone can be said to explain away 36% of the variation in Y and WEIGHT only 8%. AGE and WEIGHT together explain 37% of variation which suggests that WEIGHT doesn't contribute much over and above that obtained from AGE alone. HEIGHT does seem to add something and together with AGE accounts for almost half of the variation in Y. WEIGHT appears redundant in this model and an equation involving AGE and HEIGHT is suggested from the above. Finally, and of considerable importance, half of the variation in Y remains unaccounted for.

This simple example illustrates the potential of multiple regression in helping see the wood from the trees when there are a number of predictor variables being considered. Interactions between predictor variables can also be incorporated.

Another example illustrates that qualitative and discrete predictor variables can also be used in multiple regression, when the dependent Y variable is continuous. This is possible through use of what are called *dummy variables*:

GENDER:	G1:	$G1=1$ if male
		$G1=0$ if female
NUMBER OF CHILDREN	C1:	$C1=1$ if one child
		$C1=0$ otherwise
	C2:	$C2=1$ if two or more children
		$C2=0$ otherwise
		If $C1=0$ and $C2=0$ then person has no children
AGE GROUP	A1:	$A1=1$ if aged 65-74 years
		$A1=0$ otherwise
	A2:	$A2=1$ if aged over 75 years
		$A2=0$ if otherwise
		If $A1=0$ and $A2=0$ then person is aged under 65 years

Dummy variables take the values of zero and one. More complex qualitative and discrete variables have to be replaced by dummy variables so as to be in the form acceptable for regression modelling. Thus a discrete variable such as number of children, categorised as no children, one child, two or more children, can be replaced by two dummy variables C1 and C2.

Even a continuous variable such as age can be categorised if this is felt to be appropriate. For instance it might be felt that the variable AGE doesn't have a linear predictive effect over the whole of it's range and that simple categories of under 65, 65 to 74 years, and 75 years and over are more informative. AGE could thus be summarised by two dummy variables A1 and A2. Categorisation of a continuous predictor variable is one way of coping with a clear non-linear relationship between predictor and dependent variables.

	PREDICTOR VARIABLES	VARIATION IN Y ACCOUNTED FOR
gender	G1	10%
children	C1 and C2	6%
age	A1 and A2	25%
gender and children	G1,C1 and C2	15%
gender and age	G1,A1 and A2	29%
children and age	C1,C2,A1,A2	26%
gender,children,age	G1,C1,C2,A1,A2	30%

Thus in this example for which Y is a continuous variable the main independent predictor appears to be AGE category with GENDER allowing a little extra discrimination but not much more. After allowing for the AGE categories the CHILDREN categories account for very little extra variation in the variable Y. After the independent effects of these three variables have been accounted for 70% of the variation in Y still remains unexplained.

Logistic regression

You would consider this type of analysis when the dependent or outcome variable is binary (eg alive/dead, disease/no disease), a situation quite common in medical research, and when you have several predictor variables. There is little variability to speak of in the outcome itself other than for example the patient being alive or dead. What does vary however, and between subgroups of patients, is the proportion of patients who survive and who die.

With multiple regression it is the value of the continuous variable (eg blood pressure) which can be predicted from a set of predictor variables (eg age, sex, weight). In logistic regression it is the probability of obtaining one of the outcomes (eg the chance of being alive at one year after operation) which can be predicted. Otherwise there are many similarities in the approach to modelling.

Though both multiple and logistic regression may at first seem daunting the main messages that come out can often be simply displayed. A computer will do all the number crunching for you. Logistic regression is discussed again later in this chapter.

Other methods

Spearman's rank correlation coefficient is a non-parametric measure of the degree of association between two ordered, and hence rankable, variables. It's value lies between -1 and 1 with these two extremes indicating perfect negative and positive agreement between the ranks of the two variables. Use it in place of Pearson's coefficient when one or both variable distributions are markedly skewed and untransformable.

There are alternative methods to cope with ordinal outcomes (extension of logistic regression) and nominal outcomes (discrimination). There are methods of description (life-tables, survival curves and regression) for outcomes such as survival and recurrence of disease in longitudinal studies where subjects have been followed for differing length of time. There are also methods (cluster analysis, factor analysis) that help make sense and order out of a number of variables when there is no natural dependent or outcome variable amongst them.

There are many descriptive methods around to help you get the best out of your data. The simpler methods as described in this chapter will, in the vast majority of situations, enable you to tease out the meaningful associations from within a dataset.

Measures of Agreement

Graphical techniques

There is a subtle difference of interest between asking about the association (or correlation) of two variables and asking how well they agree.

In measuring agreement, such as between two diagnostic methods, one should expect a very high level of correlation. If the aim is to replace one method by another then the correlation has to be very good (ie above 0.95). Likewise if a measure is to be considered reliable there must be very good correlation between those who make the measurements. Good correlation however is insufficient for assessing agreement. Consider two raters (A & B) assessing patient depression on a scale ranging from 0 to 21. Each of 40 patients are assessed and graded by both raters:

Patient	1	2	3	4	5	6	7	8	9	10	11	12	13	14	15	16	17	18	19	20
Rater A	11	10	9	15	14	16	19	6	13	10	6	15	13	12	17	8	14	2	7	16
Rater B	13	8	9	16	12	15	17	8	13	11	4	17	10	16	17	7	16	6	8	9
A-B	-2	2	0	-1	2	1	2	-2	0	-1	2	-2	3	-4	0	1	-2	-4	-1	7

Patient	21	22	23	24	25	26	27	28	29	30	31	32	33	34	35	36	37	38	39	40
Rater A	5	11	13	12	8	9	12	19	18	4	6	12	12	15	10	14	15	12	9	17
Rater B	8	10	14	12	9	12	10	16	17	7	7	13	7	13	10	9	14	11	5	13
A-B	-3	1	-1	0	-1	-3	2	3	1	-3	-1	-1	5	2	0	5	1	1	4	4

Imagine a scatter plot of the above data. The vertical axis represents the assessment from rater A and the horizontal axis the assessment from rater B. Thus 40 pairs of assessments are displayed and if the two raters were in complete agreement then these 40 data points would all lie on a straight-line drawn out at 45 degrees from the origin at which the axes meet. Any disagreements, hopefully small, would be expected to be scattered evenly above and below this line. Any tendency for such discrepancies to lie mainly *above* or mainly *below* this line suggests a systematic bias between the raters.

A better way to see this graphically is to compute the differences between the two raters (A - B) and to plot these differences against their (mean) average (ie A + B / 2) (see Figure 6.5). We can see that higher average ratings do not result in larger discrepancies.

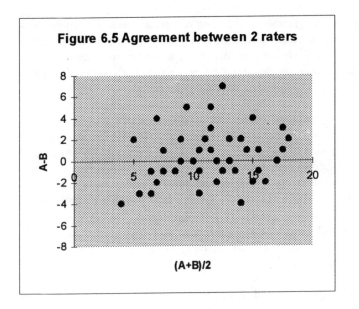

Figure 6.5 Agreement between 2 raters

Since the discrepancies display a similar scatter over the horizontal axis they can be summarised by a mean (0.43) and standard deviation (2.55) or by a median (zero) and interquartile range (-1 to +2). Alternatively a simple percentage might be enough, eg in 12 out of 40 cases (ie 30%) the discrepancy was greater than 2 units. Disagreement can also be summarised and plotted as percentage deviation. For example a discrepancy of 2 represents a 50% deviation if the average value is 4 but only a 13% deviation if the average value is 16.

The mean disagreement between raters of 0.43 estimates the bias between the raters. As this is so close to zero, the estimated level of bias between these two raters is small. Their range of disagreement can however be further defined by their mean disagreement (0.43) plus and minus twice the standard deviation of their disagreements (2.55). Thus discrepancies of between -4.7 (B>A) and 5.5 (A>B) form their 95% range of disagreement. Thus about 5% of disagreements lie beyond such boundaries. Whether these and other results are clinically acceptable would be up to you as researcher to decide.

If the disagreements had followed an inconsistent pattern over the extent of the horizontal axis then either the axis could have been subdivided and the discrepancies summarised separately, or the relationship described by regression analysis, or the whole scatterplot retained as the final summary.

The correlation coefficient (0.80 in above example) is an insufficient summary of agreement. It simply assesses the association between the two raters and we would be surprised if their ratings were unrelated. Also, the correlation would remain the same if for example one rater's values were half those reported above. Indeed in general it is possible to obtain very good correlation and very poor agreement. The above graphical approach is to be encouraged since it allows a direct assessment of the degree of discrepancy in terms of the units of measurement.

These graphical and descriptive techniques can also be used to assess agreement between two methods of measurement, by which the difference between methods is plotted against their average.

Sensitivity and specificity

Sensitivity and specificity are expressed as percentages and both depend on some valid reference measurement being available, as in this example:

A new automated non-invasive screening test to predict the presence or absence of a disease is to be assessed. Test predictions made on suitable patients are to be compared with reference biopsy results. According to biopsy findings a sample of 200 people with the disease and a sample of 300 people without the disease are selected. The new automated testings are then carried out by persons unaware of biopsy findings.

		BIOPSY FINDINGS	
		present	absent
NEW AUTOMATED TEST	present	180	60
	absent	20	240
	total	200	300

Sensitivity, in the above example, measures how well the presence of disease is predicted by a diagnostic test. The sensitivity is 180 divided by 200, that is 90 percent. Thus 90 percent of patients with the disease are appropriately diagnosed as having the disease by the new test.

Specificity measures how well the absence of disease is predicted by a diagnostic test. Above, the specificity is 240 over 300, that is 80 percent. Thus 80 percent of patients without the disease are appropriately diagnosed as not having the disease by the new test.

A sensitivity of 90% and a specificity of 80% imply errors of 10% and 20% respectively.

The false negative rate is the percentage of those people with disease who are falsely predicted as negative, ie to be disease free, by the test. The false negative rate is thus 20 over 200, that is 10 percent.

The false positive rate is the percentage of those without disease who are falsely predicted as positive, ie to have the disease, by the test. The false positive rate is 60 over 300, that is 20 percent.

Thus 10% of patients with the disease will be missed by the new test and 20% of those with no disease will be classed as having the disease. The importance of these errors will vary according to the implications of the disease and of further investigation and treatment.

A diagnostic test may give out a quantitative score and having compared the frequency distributions of scores for those with and without the disease you might be able to find a suitable cut-off score. For example:

> Score under 55 predicts disease present
>
> Score 55 and above predicts disease absent

Such a cut-off rule might carry with it a sensitivity of 90% and specificity of 80%. Varying the cut-off score will change the values of sensitivity and specificity and to observe these changes it is best to construct a graph with both the sensitivity and specificity on the vertical y-axis plotted against the cut-off value on the x-axis. The relative importance of the false positive and negative errors will help decide the most appropriate cut-off point. Any classification rule chosen in this way does however require validation in a fresh dataset (unless the cut-off is defined in advance of data collection). In other words you must try out your cut-off rule with new patients.

Positive and negative predictive values

In the examples above it is not clear what the prevalence of the disease is, and this is important because the predictive ability of a test depends upon disease prevalence in those liable to be tested. Sensitivity and specificity take no account of disease prevalence.

If the 500 patients can be regarded as a representative consecutive series drawn from the population likely to be screened then the prevalence of disease in those being tested by the new test will be 200 over 500, that is 40 percent. Should the prevalence of disease in the screened population be different than that seen in the study then allowance has to be made for this. For practical resource reasons the less common the disease under study the more likely will the reference positives and negatives be drawn as separate samples. The representativeness of separately chosen samples is an important issue especially if there are other subgroups within the intended screened population that have been omitted from the study.

Positive and negative predictive values compliment the sensitivity and specificity. If we can assume that the above 500 patients are a representative mix of the population likely to be screened (ie with a prevalence of 40%) then we can get predictive values directly from the table. Thus of 240 patients predicted to have the disease (ie test positives), 75 percent (180 of 240) actually do have the disease. Of 260 test patients predicted to be disease free (ie test negatives), then 92 percent (240 of 260) are disease free. Positive predictive values (PPV) and negative predictive values (NPV) can also be computed from the formulae below:

$$PPV = \frac{\text{sensitivity X prevalence}}{(\text{sensitivity X prevalence}) + (100\text{-specificity}) X (100\text{-prevalence})}$$

$$NPV = \frac{\text{specificity X } (100\text{-prevalence})}{(\text{specificity X } (100\text{-prevalence})) + (100\text{-sensitivity}) X (\text{prevalence})}$$

THUS:

$$PPV = \frac{90X40}{90X40 + 20X60} = 75 \text{ percent}$$

$$NPV = \frac{80X60}{80X60 + 10X40} = 92 \text{ percent}$$

Should the prevalence of disease in the screened population be different than those in the study samples then the formulae above should be used. For example with sensitivity of 90% and specificity of 80%:-

Prevalence of disease in population to be screened	Positive Predictive Value	Negative Predictive Value
10 %	33 %	99 %
20 %	53 %	97 %
30 %	66 %	95 %
40 % as above	75 %	92 %
50 %	82 %	89 %

With sensitivity and specificity held constant the lower the prevalence rate the worse the ability of the test to predict the presence of disease. Failure to acknowledge that the prevalence may well be lower than that seen between well chosen patient groups will lead to false hopes and claims about a particular diagnostic test.

Logistic regression

An alternative approach to diagnostic prediction is logistic regression. Several predictive variables, (eg automated test result, age, sex, and weight) could be looked at together and their combined predictive ability teased out. The dependent variable in this example is biopsy result (disease/no disease). The resulting logistic regression equation will allow the chance of disease to be computed for each person to be screened. For instance a man, aged 45, of 75Kg and with an automated test score of 65 might have a 94% chance of having the disease. A woman, aged 43, of 57 Kg and with a test score of 45 may only have a 13% chance of having the disease.

Any rules for prediction, derived from one dataset should be tested out in a fresh dataset. One method of doing this is to derive a prediction rule from say only 75% (randomly chosen) of the patients on whom data have been collected and to apply the rule afresh to the remaining 25%.

Kappa

The Kappa statistic relates the amount of agreement seen to the amount of agreement one might have expected by chance. Like the predictive positive and negative values the computation of Kappa's statistic is sensitive to the prevalence level. In the above example assuming 40% prevalence:

		BIOPSY FINDINGS	
		present	absent
NEW AUTOMATED TEST	present	180	60
	absent	20	240
	total	200	300

The number of patients for whom agreement between test and reference values is observed is $180+240 = 420$ which represents 84 percent of the total. The observed proportion of agreement is thus 0.84.

Even if the test values bore no relationship to the true reference values there would still be some chance agreement to be seen in the table. With an overall prevalence of disease of 40 percent (200 over 500) then one might expect 40 percent of 240 test positives (ie 96 patients) to agree with the reference biopsy positives. Likewise one might expect 60 percent of 260 test negatives (ie 156 patients) to coincide with the reference biopsy negatives. The expected chance proportion of agreement is then computed as $96+156=252$ over 500, that is 0.504 or 50 percent of patients. So even if the diagnostic test was of no use at all as a predictive measure then the above table would be expected to show agreement for about half of the patients in the study.

Kappa's statistic is computed as follows:

$$K = \frac{\text{observed proportion minus expected proportion}}{\text{one} \quad \text{minus} \quad \text{expected proportion}}$$

Thus:

$$K = \frac{0.840 - 0.504}{1.000 - 0.504} = \frac{0.336}{0.496} = 0.68$$

Clearly the formula for Kappa implies that should there be complete agreement (that is the observed proportion is 1.00) then the value of Kappa is 1.00. Also if the level of observed agreement is the same as the level expected by chance (when the test is of no predictive value) then the value of Kappa is zero. A value of Kappa of less than zero would imply a level of observed agreement less than that expected by chance. The meaning to be given to other Kappa coefficient values can be gleaned from the following:

KAPPA	INTERPRETATION	
below zero	poor	agreement
zero to 0.20	slight	agreement
0.21 to 0.40	fair	agreement
0.41 to 0.60	moderate	agreement
0.61 to 0.80	substantial	agreement
0.81 and above	almost perfect	agreement

A value of 0.68 suggests that the diagnostic test predictions substantially agree with the reference values. This taken together with a sensitivity of 90%, specificity of 80%, predictive positive and negative values of 75% and 92% respectively, helps to describe how useful the test is in predicting the presence or absence of disease.

Kappa's statistic can also be applied to ordinal, nominal and discrete data. Consider the following example in which two dental examiners each look into the mouths of 100 consecutively chosen patients. This might be done as a reliability check.

EXAMINER TWO	EXAMINER ONE number of teeth with caries			
	zero	one	two+	total
zero	31	7	1	39
one	8	22	10	40
two+	1	6	14	21
total	40	35	25	100

Kappa's statistic works out to be 0.49, indicating only a moderate level of agreement between the two examiners, and this is a disappointing finding.

Further reading (See Chapter 9 for full list of references):

Ref 1 (chpt 5, 6, 7, 15, 16)
Ref 2 (chpt 2, 3, 9, 10, 19)
Ref 5 (p188-196)
Ref 6 (p42-46)
Ref's 8, 10, 12,
14.1, 14.3, 14.4, 14.6,
15.1, 15.2, 15.7, 15.8, 15.9, 15.10,
18, 19, 22, 23

7. STATISTICAL INFERENCE & SAMPLE SIZE

There should be a clear link in your study protocol between the purpose of the study, the design plan, the variables, the analysis of data and the sample size. The quality of a study depends on careful planning, and no analysis however sophisticated will save one that has been poorly designed.

This chapter will give you a better understanding of the logic underlying tests of significance and confidence intervals. The latter certainly causes a great deal of confusion. This understanding will help. you define the role of statistical inference in your research. It will also show you how you can harness such logic to come up with a better estimate of the number of subjects you need.

A sample is of interest for what it tells about the population it represents and for a random sample the laws of probability can be taken on board in statistical analyses to assess the likely sampling variation. The larger the random sample the more accurate will any sample estimate (eg of population mean, proportion) be, and the smaller the random sampling error that will be attached to this estimate. This chapter describes two common probability distributions, the normal and binomial distributions, and explains their crucial role in statistical inference.

The representativeness of samples is a key issue in the discussion of results. For practical reasons most medical samples are unlikely to be random. However, if a sample can be considered representative then any inferences made about a population should be reasonably accurate. The extent of departure from ideal random sampling must become an important factor in the conclusions to be drawn from a study.

Normal distribution

The normal distribution is no more than a mathematical equation. When drawn the curve will always resemble a bell shape but will differ in its centre on the horizontal axis according to the value of the mean, and will differ in its peakedness/flatness according to the value of the standard deviation. The curve has two points of inflection (that is points at which the curve changes from being concave to being convex) and these are at the same distance either side of the mean. This distance, on the horizontal axis, between mean and point of inflection is the standard deviation.

So imagine a bell-shaped symmetrical curve. About two-thirds of the area under the curve lies within one standard deviation of the mean. Similarly the area under the curve within two standard deviations is about 95% of the total area. Virtually all of the area under the curve (99.8 percent) lies within 3 standard deviations of the mean.

The frequency distributions of real life data may be such that their shapes resemble that of the normal distribution curve (see discussion of mean and standard deviation in previous chapter):

You have drawn a relative frequency polygon to summarise a distribution of weights of 237 males. The mean weight is 75 kg, and the standard deviation is 8 kg.

Imagine a bell-shaped normal distribution curve drawn over this relative frequency polygon, with the shape of the curve being determined by the sample mean (75 Kg) and standard deviation (8 Kg).

If the overlap match is good then the sample mean and standard deviation are appropriate summary statistics for the frequency distribution. The theoretical properties of the normal distribution are such that you can say that about two-thirds of sample values lie within one standard deviation either side the mean, and about 95% lie within two standard deviations. Thus above, given a good overlap, then about two-thirds of male weights are between 67 Kg and 83 Kg, and about 95% are between 59 Kg and 91 kg.

If a sample frequency distribution shows a pronounced skewness then it is not so meaningful to compute the values of the sample mean and standard deviation. The normal distribution curve determined by these values will be bell-shaped and symmetrical and will be unlike the shape of the skewed distribution. Some transformation of the data (eg square-root, logarithm, reciprocal) such that the transformed scale provides a good approximation may be the answer. Then the mean and standard deviation in the transformed scale can be quoted as summary statistics for the distribution. If no suitable transformation is possible then summary by the median and percentile ranges is indicated.

Practical assessment of normal approximation

1. Look at the shape of the frequency distribution. Does it look symmetrical? Draw a box & whisker plot. If it is grossly skewed can the variable be transformed so that the transformed distribution looks symmetrical?

2. Compute the sample mean and standard deviation. Check to see if about two-thirds of the data do fall within one standard deviation of the mean and that about 95% fall within about two standard deviations.

3. Draw a normal plot using a special type of graph paper (or tell your computer to do so). The horizontal axis represents the scale of measurement of the variable (eg weight). The vertical axis is scaled unevenly from 0% to 100% in such a way that the cumulative relative frequency plot for a normally distributed variable would show itself on the plot as a straight line. Deviations from a straight line suggest non-normality.

Distribution of the sample mean

Imagine you have a large sampling frame of patients, listed by surname:

Suppose you take a random sample of 100 adult patients from the sampling frame and you measure their heights. You compute the mean height (175 cms) and standard deviation of heights (9cms) for the sample.

Then starting again from the full list of names you select another random sample of 100 patients (this second sample might include some patients chosen the first time) and measure their heights. You compute the sample mean (173 cms) and standard deviation (8cms). Imagine repeating this process lots of times.

You would end up with lots of independently chosen random samples of 100 patients. For each sample you would have measured 100 heights, and computed a mean and a standard deviation. You would thus have lots of sample mean heights each providing an estimate of the mean height of the sampling frame population. Thus you can imagine a sampling distribution of means, that is the distribution of sample means you would get if this process were to be repeated many times. You can also imagine a mean and standard deviation of these sample means.

This distribution of sample means will in fact approximate to a normal distribution the shape of which can be described by the mean and standard deviation of the sample means. [Note: This approximation happens whether or not the distribution of population heights resembles a normal distribution. The greater the skewness in the distribution of population heights the greater the sample size that is required for the sampling distribution of the mean to approach normality.]

To avoid confusion between the standard deviation of a set of individual measurements in a single sample and the standard deviation of a set of sample means the latter is called the standard error (SE) of the mean. (The SE always refers to the estimate of a population parameter).

In the usual research situation one has to make do with a single sample, and the population mean and standard deviation are unknown. How close to the true population mean will the single sample mean be? The precision of a sample mean is estimated by the standard error of the mean, computed as follows:

$$\text{Standard Error of Mean (SEM)} = \frac{\text{sample standard deviation}}{\text{square root of sample size}}$$

Confidence interval

The sample mean plus and minus twice the standard error of the mean gives the 95 percent confidence interval for the mean and describes a range of possible true mean values (for the population) consistent with the sample data obtained.

In a random sample of size 100 suppose the mean height was 171 cms and the standard deviation was 8 cms, and the frequency distribution of heights approximates to a normal distribution. About two-thirds of heights are between 163 and 179 cms and about 95% are between 155 and 187 cms.

The standard error of the mean is 8cms/$\sqrt{100}$ = 0.8 cms. Thus the 95 percent confidence interval for the mean is 171 cms plus or minus twice the standard error, that is from 169.4 to 172.6 cms. There is therefore 95 percent confidence that this range from 169.4 to 172.6 cms includes the true population mean height.

The normal distribution occupies a central role in the techniques of statistical inference. The 95 percent confidence interval for a population mean is given by the sample mean plus & minus twice the standard error of the mean. Likewise the 95 percent confidence interval for the difference between two means is given by the sample difference between means plus & minus twice the standard error of the difference between means. The symmetry of the confidence interval follows from the assumption that the sampling distributions of the means, and difference between means, are normally distributed.

Binomial distribution

The sampling distribution of a proportion is the binomial distribution. This in turn for large samples can be approximated by the normal distribution.

The prevalence of hypertension in a very large population is already known to be 35%. Suppose you now select a random sample of 400 from this population. The number of people in your sample with hypertension is found to be 112, that is 28% (or 0.28 as a proportion).

Suppose you then choose another random sample of 400 from the population. The number of people with hypertension is now 132, that is 33% (or 0.33 as a proportion).

Suppose you continue to take random samples of 400 in this manner and each time you record the proportion of people who have hypertension.

Each sample proportion provides an estimate of the population, and you can imagine a distribution of sample proportions (0.28, 0.33 etc). This distribution of sample proportions will take on the shape of the binomial distribution determined by values of $p = 0.35$ and $n = 400$.

In fact the bigger the sample size then, with repeated sampling, the sooner the shape of the binomial probability distribution approximates the shape of the normal distribution. The closer that p is to 0.5 then the quicker this happens. This approximation to a normal distribution is important because for large samples (a rough guide to this is that np and n(1-p) are both more than five) the precision of the proportion can be estimated by the following:

---

standard error(of proportion) = square root of $\{ p(1-p)/n \}$

Confidence interval

In the usual research setting the best estimate of the population prevalence will be the prevalence obtained in a single random sample drawn from that population. The estimate of standard error is obtained by substituting the sample proportion into the above equation:

In a random sample of 400 people 32% were hypertensive.
Thus n=400, p=0.32

The estimate of standard error is $\sqrt{[(0.32 \times 0.68)/400]} = 0.023$, ie 2.3%.

Note that both np and n(1-p) exceed five, and the normal approximation applies.

The 95 percent confidence interval for the prevalence of disease is computed as sample prevalence (0.32) plus & minus twice the standard error of the proportion (2 times 0.023), ie from 0.274 to 0.366, that is between about 27% and 37%. Thus from this single sample you would have about 95% confidence that the interval 27% to 37% includes the population prevalence of hypertension.

The 99 percent confidence interval uses the multiplier 2.6 rather then 2. Thus the 99 percent confidence interval for the population prevalence is between 26% and 38%.

Example to illustrate the meaning of a confidence interval

Suppose the true population prevalence of hypertension was known to be 35%. In reality you wouldn't bother with a study if you already knew this. For this example though we use this knowledge to examine the accuracy of the sample prevalence and of the calculated 95% confidence interval in estimating the population prevalence.

The population comprises a large number of people of whom 35% have hypertension. A random sample of 400 people was taken and the proportion with hypertension recorded. The 95 and 99 percent confidence intervals were also computed. This process was repeated 200 times. Think of these as 200 different studies, from which the results are summarised below:

Sample prevalence	Number of random samples	Approx 95% CI for population prevalence	Approx 99% CI for population prevalence
27%	1	22% to 32%	21% to 33%
29%	2	24% to 34%	23% to 35%
30%	1	25% to 35%	24% to 36%
31%	11	26% to 36%	25% to 37%
32%	15	27% to 37%	26% to 38%
33%	24	28% to 38%	27% to 39%
34%	26	29% to 39%	28% to 40%
35%	36	30% to 40%	29% to 41%
36%	26	31% to 41%	30% to 42%
37%	22	32% to 42%	31% to 43%
38%	19	33% to 43%	32% to 44%
39%	10	34% to 44%	33% to 45%
40%	4	35% to 45%	34% to 46%
41%	1	36% to 46%	35% to 47%
42%	2	37% to 47%	36% to 48%
total	200		

Which of these 200 studies would have been yours? You might have been unlucky in that your (random) sample prevalence was 42% with 95% confidence interval of 37% to 47%. Thus you might have concluded that the best estimate of prevalence in the larger population was 42% but that with 95% confidence the true prevalence lay within the range 37% to 47%.

However, if you look at the 95% confidence intervals for the above 200 studies only in 6 instances did the interval fail to include the true prevalence rate of 35%. Put another way 97% of the study confidence intervals actually did include the true prevalence. Thus in your single study you can feel reasonably happy that your single confidence interval will include the true prevalence. In general when computing the 95% confidence interval you would expect, from the long run of repeated studies, that 95 out of 100 study confidence intervals would include the true prevalence.

Only in 3 instances (1.5%) did the 99% confidence interval exclude the true prevalence rate of 35%. In the long run of repeated studies you would expect that 99 out of 100 study confidence intervals to include the true prevalence.

Tests of statistical significance, and statistical power

Tests of significance

In school geometry one used to state an hypothesis, prove it to be nonsense and hence conclude the alternative hypothesis to be true. With statistical testing the degree to which a stated (null) hypothesis can be considered nonsensical is based on a probability value. The stages in significance testing are:-

SUPPOSITION (NULL HYPOTHESIS)	eg. no difference between boys and girls in prevalence of dental decay
OBSERVATION	collect data and observe the difference in prevalence between boys and girls (eg boys=20%, girls=15%)
REASONING	is data consistent with supposition?

We have seen that probability samples are liable to random error and in the process of reasoning from a test of significance we ask how likely are we to observe differences at least as extreme as those observed if the null hypothesis were really true. This is measured by a probability value and for example $P=0.05$ represents a 5% chance of observing data at least as extreme as those collected if the null hypothesis were really true.

A legal analogy would be that one is assumed innocent until proven guilty. The quality of prosecution evidence will vary from case to case. Sometimes the evidence is so strongly stacked against the defendant that it is felt the defendant must be guilty, that is the possibility of innocence is rejected. At other times it might be felt that the prosecution evidence lacks weight and could easily be consistent with a null or working hypothesis of the defendant being innocent.

This legal analogy is a reasonable one since decision making underlies the whole approach to significance testing. In court a decision has finally to be arrived at on the basis of evidence presented to it and there is no watertight guarantee to ensure that every such decision will be without error. The errors in decision making are known as type 1 and type 2 errors:

Type 1 error: In significance testing a null hypothesis might be rejected when by chance a rare occurrence has been observed in a sample and when the null hypothesis is true. In court an innocent person might be considered guilty.

Type 2 error: Alternatively when the null hypothesis is actually false the sample data might be considered consistent with the null hypothesis. In court a guilty person is considered innocent.

The assessment of evidence against a null hypothesis is very much a matter of opinion. Probability values of $P=0.05$ and $P=0.01$ are commonly used as convenient yardsticks to reject the null hypothesis. Such 5% and 1% yardsticks are thus taken as dividing lines between statistical significance and non-significance.

Suppose the P value derived for the test of significance above between boys and girls was $P=0.03$.

You might then conclude that if the null hypothesis (of no difference in prevalence between boys and girls) were really true then the chances of observing the difference obtained (or a difference more extreme) is only 3%.

Since this chance seems quite low, and in particular P is less than 5%, then you might feel that the data are not consistent with the null hypothesis.

Hence you would conclude that there probably is a difference between boys and girls in the prevalence of dental decay. You could however be making a mistake with this conclusion. It is possible that this study result could have come about by chance, a 3% chance assuming that the null hypothesis of no difference were actually true. The chance of making a type-one error is thus 3 %.

Many researchers seem unnecessarily obsessed with tests of statistical significance and achieving statistical significance at the 5% level of significance (ie $P < 0.05$) has unfortunately become their pot of gold at the end of the rainbow. $P = 0.04$ becomes acceptable and worthy of publication whilst $P = 0.06$ is detestable (whereas these P values are virtually indistinguishable in the weight of evidence against the null hypothesis). It is better to record the actual probability value itself, possible with computer analyses, eg $P = 0.23$ and interpret accordingly. Clearly $P = 0.06$ is stronger evidence for rejecting the null hypothesis than $P = 0.23$ but all too often one might see them lumped together under the general umbrella of "statistically non-significant $P > 0.05$" or just "NS" a shorthand for non-significance. The reporting of probability values in tests of significance would allow other people greater freedom in interpreting your results.

Statistical testing can introduce a false dichotomy of thinking, through an over-concern with probability values (or P values). Results that when summarised look interesting might then be dismissed as unimportant because of a "statistically non-significant" test of significance, a small sample size often being overlooked in this process of dismissal. The weakness of the test of significance is that it centres merely on whether some effect to be tested can be regarded as statistically significant. In no way does it relate to the likely size of that effect, which is possible with confidence intervals. For example how large could the difference in prevalence of dental decay between boys and girls be? The test of significance merely tests whether no difference is one possible explanation.

The most commonly used tests of significance are shown below. Many statistical textbooks describe these in detail and it is not the intention here to do likewise. Parametric tests make various assumptions about the shape of frequency distributions and are the tests of choice if these assumptions can be met. Equality of the population standard deviations in the groups to be compared is one assumption. Another assumption is that of normality. If the frequency distributions are severely skewed and cannot (even in a transformed scale) be assumed normal then a non-parametric approach should be considered. Small to moderate departures from a normal distribution can be safely ignored but if in doubt then try both parametric and non-parametric methods.

CONTINUOUS VARIABLE: (choose parametric or non-parametric test)
DISCRETE VARIABLE: (choose non-parametric or parametric test),
ORDERED CATEGORY VARIABLE: (choose non-parametric test):

1. Comparison of two groups: unrelated or independent data

Parametric:-   Two sample t-test
Non-parametric:-   Wilcoxon rank sum test
                      Mann-Whitney U test (identical results to Wilcoxon)

2. Comparison of three or more groups: unrelated or independent data

Parametric:-   One way analysis of variance (ANOVA)
Non-parametric:-   Kruskal-Wallis test

3. Comparison of two groups: related or paired data

Parametric:-   Paired t-test
Non-parametric:-   Wilcoxon matched pairs test

4. Comparison of three or more groups: related or paired data

Parametric:-   Two way analysis of variance
Non-parametric:-   Friedman's test

CATEGORICAL VARIABLE:

1. Comparison of two or more groups: unrelated or independent data

The chi-squared test is appropriate for the comparison of proportions between groups. The test is non-parametric.

2. Comparison of two groups: related or paired data

                      McNemar's test.

Statistical power

To conclude that data are consistent with a null hypothesis doesn't rule out the possibility that the null hypothesis is wrong, in other words you can make a Type 2 error. Some of the alternative conclusions might well be of major clinical importance. If the size of sample is small then the sample data will be consistent with a wide range of conclusions. A wide confidence interval, irrespective of whether or not a statistically significant result from a significance test is found, points to a lack of information and is a warning against the over-interpretation of results from small studies.

Statistical power refers to the ability of a statistical test to lead to a rejection of a null hypothesis when the null hypothesis is false.

Suppose drug A actually improves patient outcome by 10% over that achieved by drug B.

This 10% difference represents the least effect really worth knowing about.

The experiment should be designed so that a test of statistical significance (chi-squared test) would have a very good chance (eg 80% power) of achieving a statistically significant result (eg $p < 0.05$).

A study with 80% power carries with it a 20% chance of making a type 2 error.

Would you want your study to miss the smallest clinically worthwhile difference should it exist? Unfortunately many experiments fail even to have 50% power to detect quite sizeable (not minimum) differences between groups. The danger then is in reporting a statistically non-significant difference, and concluding from this that no meaningful difference exists, when in fact an important difference could exist.

Statistical power is a concept inevitably bound up with tests of significance and is, by the predominance of small studies, poorly understood. Statements about the power of statistical tests to be used, and relevant to this, the minimum differences worth knowing about rarely appear in the statistical methods sections of published reports. If you want to use statistical tests of significance you should make a point of stating the required statistical power in your protocol. As you shall soon see this will lead you into estimating a sample size big enough to satisfy your requirements.

Sample size

Your protocol should state how many subjects are needed and why this number is necessary. Having too few subjects means that sample estimates will be unreliable, whilst a sample far too big for the purpose will squander resources. Compute the sample size required to give good answers to your most important questions. This chapter considers the most common parameters, and avoids numerical complexity as much as possible:

Common parameters:

Mean
Proportion
Difference between means
Difference between proportions

It must be said that sample size forecasting is at best an inexact science being dependent on assumptions, speculations and requirements. One assumption you make is of random sampling. The underlying idea though is to get a feel for the right order of magnitude and to avoid enrolling far too few or far too many subjects.

You want your results to be precise, and the key to sample size estimation is the standard error. The smaller the standard error the narrower the confidence interval, and the more precise is your estimate of the population parameter (eg difference between two means). Also the smaller the standard error the higher the statistical power of a test of significance, and the lower the chance of making a type 2 error (eg of not finding a meaningful difference between means when in reality a meaningful difference does exist).

Increasing the sample size decreases the standard error. It is up to you to define your requirements and then to study enough subjects so that you can get the precision you desire. In analysis this careful planning will show up as small standard errors, narrow confidence intervals and tests of significance with lots of power.

You can compute sample sizes either through estimation and the use of confidence intervals or through statistical power and the use of tests of significance.

Sample size and estimation

You should decide an acceptable width of the confidence interval you wish to compute in your analysis. Too wide and the results will lack precision, too tight and you waste resources. The method of computation is best explained by a couple of examples highlighting the proportion and the mean, though the basic logic can be extended to other parameters:

1. **Proportion**:

$$SE = \text{Standard Error} = \sqrt{(p(1-p)/n)}$$

$$95\% \text{ CI} = 95\% \text{ Confidence interval} = p \pm 2SE$$

p is the sample proportion.
n is the sample size.

Suppose you are planning a study to determine the prevalence of diabetes in a large "at-risk" population of adults aged 45 years and over. You decide you want an estimate of prevalence to be accurate to within $\pm 5\%$. Thus you have set the half-width of the confidence interval to 5%. This half-width is equivalent to twice the standard error, and hence you have set the required standard error to be 2.5% or 0.025 as a proportion. Thus using the above equation for the standard error:

$$0.025 = \sqrt{((p(1-p)/n))}$$

$$\text{ie } n = p(1-p)/(0.025)^2$$

$$\text{ie } n = p(1-p)/(0.000625)$$

You may have some idea of the likely prevalence, based perhaps on your literature review or on pilot work. For example suppose you expected a prevalence of diabetes of about 20%. Substitute the values p=0.15 & p=0.25 into the above equation to obtain values for n:

p=0.15	n = (0.15)(0.85)/(0.000625)	= 204
p=0.20	n = (0.2)(0.8)/(0.000625)	= 256
p=0.25	n = (0.25)(0.75)/(0.000625)	= 300

From these computations you would conclude that about 300 subjects should be studied to give you the required precision.

2. **Mean**:

SE $\quad$ = Standard Error = $SD/\sqrt{n}$

95% CI $\quad$ = 95% Confidence Interval $\quad$ = $\quad$ mean $\pm$ 2SE

SD is the sample Standard Deviation
n is the sample size

Suppose you are planning a study of hypertension in a large population of adults aged 45 years and over. As part of the study you wish to obtain an estimate of mean systolic blood pressure accurate to within about 2.5 mmHg. Thus you have set the half-width of the confidence interval to 2.5 mmHg. This half-width is equivalent to twice the standard error, and hence you have set the required standard error to be 1.25 mmHg. Thus using the above equation for the standard error:

1.25 = $SD/\sqrt{n}$

ie n $= SD^2/(1.25)^2$

ie n $= SD^2/1.5625$

You may have some idea of the likely value of the standard deviation, based perhaps on your literature review or on pilot work. Suppose you expect a standard deviation of about 20. Substitute the values SD=15 and SD=25 into the above equation to obtain values of n:

SD = 15 mmHg	n = 225/1.5625 = 144
SD = 20 mmHg	n = 400/1.5625 = 256
SD = 25 mmHg	n = 625/1.5625 = 400

From these computations you would conclude that about 400 subjects should be studied to give you the required precision. As you can see from these computations the more variable the data the more subjects you need to study to achieve a required level of precision in your analysis.

Sample size and statistical power

You should decide an acceptable power of the test of significance you wish to use in your analysis, and the kind of differences between groups that you think are worth detecting. These are the sort of questions a statistician would ask of you. Make sure your study has at least an 80% chance of unearthing a meaningful difference should one really exist. The method of sample size computation is best explained by a couple of examples highlighting the difference between two proportions and the difference between two means, though the approach can be extended to the comparison of other parameters:

1. **Difference between two proportions:**

Null Hypothesis : no difference between two population proportions.

p_1 & p_2 are the sample proportions.
n is the number of patients in each group.

Suppose you are planning a randomized clinical trial to evaluate a new drug. The new drug is to be compared with an existing commonly used drug, and the main outcome is full recovery from the disease under study. The appropriate statistical test is the chi-squared test.

You should decide the minimum level of improvement between the drugs on trial that you feel is of clinical value. Suppose considerable experience with the existing treatment suggests a full recovery rate of about 20% and that you decide a difference of 10% or more in full recovery rates between drugs shouldn't be missed.

Thus if there really was a difference of 10% then you would want the study chi-squared test to show a statistically significant result (ie $P < 0.05$). The degree of certainty with which the study will yield a statistically significant result is the power, and a power of 80% or more is desirable. Sample sizes can be obtained from the following formulae:

For 50% power and $P < 0.05$ then:
$$n = 4[p_1(1-p_1)+p_2(1-p_2)]/(p_1-p_2)^2 \text{ per group}$$

For 80% power and $P < 0.05$ then:
$$n = 8[p_1(1-p_1)+p_2(1-p_2)]/(p_1-p_2)^2 \text{ per group}$$

For 90% power and $P < 0.05$ then:
$$n = 11[p_1(1-p_1)+p_2(1-p_2)]/(p_1-p_2)^2 \text{ per group}$$

p_1 is the proportion of patients taking the existing drug who fully recover.
p_2 is the proportion of patients taking the new drug and who fully recover.

Thus if a 20% recovery rate is expected for the existing drug (ie $p_1=0.20$) and if an improvement on the new treatment of 10% or more should not be missed (ie $p_2=0.30$) then the formula (for 80% power & $P<0.05$) gives:

For 80% power and $P<0.05$:

$$n = 8[(0.20)(0.80) + (0.30)(0.70)]/(0.20-0.30)^2$$
$$= 8[0.16 + 0.21]/(0.1)^2$$
$$= 8[0.37]/0.01$$
$$= 296 \text{ patients per group}$$

So about 300 patients per group would be required for the study to have 80% power, ie 600 patients in all. Note that a study with fewer than 150 patients per group would have less than a 50% chance of showing a statistically significant result (ie $P<0.05$ in a chi-squared test) if there was a difference of 10% in full-recovery rates between the two drugs.

2. Difference between two means:

Null Hypothesis : no difference between two population means.

$Mean_1$ & $Mean_2$ are the sample means.
n is the number of patients in each group.

Suppose you are planning a clinical trial to compare two dietary treatments for eczema. The main outcome is a measure of the amount of body area affected by eczema. Assessments are made before randomization and again after the treatment period. The outcome to be compared between diets A and B is the change in body area score. The appropriate parametric statistical test is the unpaired t-test.

You should decide the minimum level of improvement, between the diets on trial, that you feel is of clinical value. From previous experience in using one of these diets (diet A) you expect the mean eczema body area score will improve about 30 units over the treatment period. Experience also suggests considerable variation in individual changes over time, measured by a standard deviation of changes of about 35 units.

Suppose you decide that a treatment difference between diets of 10 units or more is important for the research to detect. For example if the mean change in body area score with diet A is 30 units and if the mean change in body area score with diet B is 40 units, then there is a treatment difference between diets of 10 units. A 10 unit mean difference is thus the minimum you think is clinically worth knowing about.

If there really was a difference of this magnitude then you would want the t-test to show a statistically significant result (ie $P < 0.05$) when the data were analysed. The degree of certainty with which the study will yield a statistically significant result is the power, and a power of 80% or more is desirable. Sample sizes can be obtained from the following formulae:

For 50% power and $P < 0.05$ then:
$$n = 8SD^2/(Mean_1 - Mean_2)^2 \text{ per group}$$

For 80% power and $P < 0.05$ then:
$$n = 16SD^2/(Mean_1 - Mean_2)^2 \text{ per group}$$

For 90% power and $P < 0.05$ then:
$$n = 21SD^2/(Mean_1 - Mean_2)^2 \text{ per group}$$

SD is the Standard Deviation, assumed to be the same for both groups.

$(Mean_1 - Mean_2)$ is the minimum treatment difference worth knowing about.

Thus if the minimum treatment difference is $(Mean_1-Mean_2)$ $=10$ units, and the standard deviation in each group is 35 units, then:

Power of 80% and $P < 0.05$:

$n \quad = 16(35)^2/(10)^2$
$= 16(1225)/100$
$= 196$ patients per group.

Putting in the values of SD=30 and SD=40 as alternative guesses for the standard deviation gives 144 and 256 patients per group respectively. From these computations you would conclude that about 200-250 patients should be studied on each diet to give you 80% power. As you can see from these computations the more variable the data the more subjects you need to study to achieve a required level of power in your analysis.

A few final thoughts:

1. A clinical trial was chosen as the setting for the last two examples. The same reasoning about sample size can also be applied in any situation when you wish to make a comparison between two groups, such as between cases and controls or when comparing observational cohort exposure subgroups.

2. Hopefully the computed sample sizes will fall within your envisaged scale of operation. Sadly the figures often imply a research workload far in excess of that anticipated. The consequences then are that either:

a) You give up.
b) You recruit more subjects by increasing the length of your study.
c) You recruit more subjects by increasing the number of participating centres, doctors and so forth.
d) You water down your precision criteria.

There is the great temptation to head for the last category, for example to choose a lower power or to allow a more relaxed minimum worthwhile difference. Be very wary of doing this. Consider options b. and c., and even a.. Should you invest time, effort & resources into a study that has only a very slim chance of discovering something worthwhile?

3. There is a temptation to analyse data in all ways possible, looking within many subgroups and making many comparisons. Such torture usually confesses something and it is reasonable to report such findings but these do not carry the weight of findings that confirm or refute hypotheses generated at the beginning of a study. Remember that prior speculation as to future outcome is the basis on which good research is rooted and that the most important analyses relate to the questions posed at the design stage of the project. Findings from data torture require validation in a fresh study.

4. Minor changes in the selection or exclusion criteria (and thus affecting the variability of data) could have an important effect on the width of confidence intervals, and on the tests of significance. Researchers often exclude certain subgroups in an effort to obtain more homogeneous samples. If the study population is made too narrow then generalisation of results will run into problems of credibility. To serve the purpose of wide generalisation then as full a range of subjects as possible should be included.

5. As discussed in chapter 4 many researchers do not take, and often cannot possibly take, random samples and even the taking of a sample by probabilistic methods doesn't always produce a random sample. At best they might claim to have representative samples:

In a general practice diabetes survey those people registered and aged 40 or over comprised the study population and a sample of 400 was chosen by random methods and invited for screening.

Unfortunately only 200 of these people turned up for screening and in these a prevalence rate of 10% was noted.

How reasonable is it to infer from this sample result through a confidence interval to the whole population aged 40 or over and registered with the practice? The answer is that it seems unreasonable. The possibility of non-random bias in the 50% who failed to respond is too great for direct generalisation. The confidence interval if computed might more realistically relate to the population who would be likely to respond to an invitation for screening. In this example a random sample of the non-responders could be chased in order to provide an estimate of the likely bias involved in non-response.

As a general policy, however, it is reasonable to compute confidence intervals whether or not you feel you have a random sample from your target group. Quite what the sample represents may however be unclear and it is the art of discussion to combine information from the confidence interval with non-statistical considerations to produce an overall conclusion.

Likewise the same reasoning would apply to tests of significance. It is reasonable to do them but then you need to bring in non-statistical considerations to make overall sense of the results.

The saving grace of randomized controlled trials, for which the source of the pre-randomization sample is usually convenience, lies in the process of random allocation. Randomization ensures the overall validity of calculating confidence intervals and doing tests of significance. However, whatever final interpretations are made regarding differences between interventions they strictly apply at best to the study population.

6. You will have noticed the clear separation between description and statistical inference. As a general policy it makes sense to do this second phase of statistical inference but to bear in mind that any direct inference from sample to target population could be very much in error if a major source of sampling error is non-random.

I hope that you can now put together a well balanced and well reasoned protocol, and that your research goes well. If you haven't already done so, now is the time you should pay that overdue visit to your friendly statistician to talk over all aspects of the study design. Any comments about this book are gratefully received, via the publishers.

Further reading (See Chapter 9 for full list of references):

Ref 1 (chpt 9 to 14, 24, 25)
Ref 2 (chpt 4 to 7, 12, 14, 26)
Ref 5 (chpt 9, 13.2, 13.3)
Ref's 8, 9, 10,
14.2, 14.5, 15.3, 15.4, 15.5, 15.6,
16, 20, 21, 26, 29, 30, 35, 36, 38, 39,

8. CHECK LIST FOR EVALUATING RESEARCH PROTOCOLS

This can be used by another person to assess your protocol, or by you to assess the protocols of others. Answer each as **Yes**, **No** or **Unclear**

1. Title

Does the title adequately summarise the content of the research protocol?

2. Statement of problem.

a. Is the research problem clearly stated?
b. Is it clear how the idea for research came about?
c. Is the study original in concept?

3. Significance of research. (Who will benefit?)

If achieved will the study be of benefit to the Health Service?

4. Research Background.

a. Are all important aspects of the problem clearly stated?
b. Are all pertinent findings from the literature appropriately reviewed, and their relevance to the problem stated?

5. Purpose of Research.

a. Is the purpose clearly defined and does it derive directly from the statement of the problem?
b. Is the purpose realistic and relevant?
c. Does the purpose make clear the data that will need to be collected?
d. Does the purpose make clear the populations that will be studied?

6. Hypotheses and Speculation as to Outcome of Research

a. Are expectations from the research clearly expressed?
b. Do hypotheses derive directly from the statement of the problem?
c. Is it clear what data will need to be collected to confirm or refute the stated expectations?

7. Design of Study

a. Are the data to be collected described?
b. Are the data to be collected relevant to the purpose of the research?
c. Are important data omitted?

d. Are the procedures for data measurement given in detail?
e. Will the data be reliable?
f. Will the data be valid?

g. Is the sampling methodology fully described?
h. Does the study require a control group?
i. Does the protocol describe a control group?

j. Is the protocol control group appropriate?
k. Are exclusion criteria for subjects clearly defined?
l. Will a log or diary of excluded subjects be kept?

m. Is there a satisfactory statement of the source of subjects (eg case and controls)?
n. Will the sample(s) be representative of the relevant population(s)?
o. Are the number of subjects to be studied stated?

p. Is there a clear justification for the number of subjects to be studied?
q. Are the stated number of subjects adequate?
r. Are the stated number of subjects likely to be available for study?

s. Has the plan for analysis been fully described?
t. Is the plan for analysis appropriate?
u. Is a pilot study necessary?

v. Will a pilot study be done?
w. Is an adequate description given of what will be done in the pilot study?
x. Are there any outstanding ethical issues?

y. Is the methodological design of the study consistent with it's purpose?
z. Overall has the design plan been well thought out?

8. Staff, Facilities and Resources

a. Will the grades of staff who carry out the study be suitable for the research in question?
b. Is there evidence (eg past record) that named researchers can fulfil the tasks required of them?
c. Is there to be a steering group to oversee the progress of the project?

d. Will the available or planned facilities, equipment
and other resources be adequate?
e. Is the funding for the research realistic?
f. Do the potential benefits from the research warrant the requested funds?
g. If the research depends on permission from others being given have necessary steps been taken to secure their support and agreement?

9. Overall

a. Is there a clear link running through the whole protocol from the statement of problem to the type of study design, the variables to be measured, and the intended mode of analysis?
b. Has the proposal generally been well thought out?
c. Is the study acceptable in its present form?
d. If the study is not acceptable in its present
form can it be revised so that it becomes acceptable?

10. Any additional comments? Give details.

9. FURTHER READING

Each book or journal article below is given a reference number. These references (as numbers) can be found at the end of chapters 1 to 7 as suggestions for further reading.

BOOKS:

1. Bradford-Hill Sir A. *A short textbook of medical statistics*. Hodder and Stoughton, Sevenoaks, Kent 1984.
2. Kirkwood BR. *Essentials of medical statistics*. Blackwell, Oxford. 1988.
3. Lilienfeld AM, Lilienfeld DE. *Foundations of epidemiology*. Oxford University Press 1980
4. Meddis R. *Statistical handbook for non-statisticians*. McGraw-Hill, Maidenhead, Berkshire 1975.
5. Pocock SJ. *Clinical trials: a practical approach*. Wiley, Chichester 1983.
6. Rose G, Barker DJP. *Epidemiology for the uninitiated*. British Medical Association, London 1986.
7. Stuart A. *The ideas of sampling*. Monograph No. 4, Griffen and Company, High Wycombe 1984

ARTICLES: Many of these are from accessible journals:

8. Altman DG. Statistics in medical journals. *Statistics in Medicine* 1982;**1**:59-71.
9. Altman DG, Gardner MJ Calculating confidence intervals for regression and correlation. *BMJ* 1988 ;**296**:1238-1242.
10. Altman DG, Gore SM, Gardner MJ, Pocock SJ. Statistical guidelines for contributors to medical journals. *BMJ* 1983;**286**:1489-1493.
11. Barker KN. Data Collection Techniques: Observation. *American Journal of Hospital Pharmacy* 1980;**37**:1235-43.
12. Bland JM, Altman DG. Statistical methods for assessing agreement between two methods of clinical measurement. *Lancet* 1986:307-310.
13. Bork CE, Francis JB. Developing Effective Questionnaires. *Physical Therapy* 1985;**65**:907-911
14. Brown RA, Swanson Beck J. Statistics on microcomputers: a non-algebraic guide to their appropriate use in biomedical research and pathology laboratory practice. A series of six articles. *Journal of Clinical Pathology:*
    1. Data handling and preliminary analysis. 1988;**41**:1033-1038.
    2. Confidence intervals and significance tests. 1988;**41**:1148-1154.
    3. ANOVA and distribution-free methods. 1988;**41**:1256-1262.
    4. Correlation and regression. 1989;**42**:4-12.
    5. Analysis of categorical data. 1989;**42**:117-122.
    6. Statistical methods for diagnostic tests. 1989;**42**:225-230.
15. Bulman JS, Osborn JF. Statistics in Dentistry. *British Dental Journal:*1989
    1. Descriptive statistics. **166**:51-54.
    2. Simple summary calculations. **166**:87-90.
    3. Probability and sampling. **166**:132-135.
    4. Significance tests. **166**:178-180.
    5. Significance tests: Part 2. **166**:218-221.
    6. Significance tests: part 3. **166**:261-264.
    7. Analysing the association between two variables. **166**:303-307.

8. Comparison of several groups. **166**:341-343.

9. Measuring diagnostic consistency. **166**:377-381.

10. Statistical Analysis: the future. **166**:417-419.

16. Campbell MJ, Gardner MJ. Calculating confidence intervals for some non-parametric analyses. *BMJ* 1988;**296**:1454-1456.

17. Cancer Research Campaign Working Party in Breast Conservation. Informed consent: ethical, legal, and medical implications for doctors and patients who participate in randomized clinical trials. *BMJ* 1983;**286**:1117-21.

18. Cohen JA coefficient of agreement for nominal scales. *Educ Psychol Measurement* 1960;**20**:37-46.

19. Cohen J. Weighted kappa: Nominal scale agreement with provision for scaled disagreement or partial credit. *Psychological Bulletin* 1968;**70**:213-20.

20. Gardner MJ, Altman DG. Confidence intervals rather than P values: estimation rather than hypothesis testing. *BMJ* 1986;**292**:746-750.

21. Glantz SA. Biostatistics: How to detect, correct and prevent errors in the medical literature. *Circulation* 1980;**61**:1-7.

22. Godrey KAM. Simple linear regression in medical research. *New England Journal of Medicine* 1985;**313**:1629-1636.

23. Jacobsen BS. Know thy data. *Nursing Research* 1981;**30**:254-255.

24. Jang R. General Purpose of Research Designs. *American Journal of Hospital Pharmacy* 1980;**37**:398-403.

25. Leading article. Meta-analysis. *British Journal of Surgery* 1990: **77**, 243-4.

26. Machin D, Gardner MJ. Calculating confidence intervals for survival time analyses. *BMJ* 1988;**296**:1369-1371.

27. Manasse HR Jr, Lambert RL. Types of Research: A Synopsis of the Major Categories and Data Collection Methods. *American Journal of Hospital Pharmacy* 1980;**37**:694-701.

28. Meier P. Statistics and medical experimentation. *Biometrics* 1975;**31**:511-29

29. Meijer WS, Schmitz PIM, Jeekel J. Meta-analysis of randomized contolled clinical trials of antibiotic prophylaxis in biliary tract surgery. *British Journal of Surgery* 1990;**77**:283-290.

30. Morris JA, Gardner MJ. Calculating confidence intervals for relative risks (odds ratios) and standardised ratios and rates. *BMJ* 1988;**296**:1313-1316.

31. Moses LE. Statistical concepts fundamental to investigations. *New England Journal of Medicine* 1985;**312**:890-897.

32. Nelson AA Jr. Research Design: Measurement, Reliability, and Validity. *American Journal of Hospital Pharmacy* 1980;**37**:851-7.

33. Pathak DS, Meinhold JM, Fisher DJ. Research Design: Sampling Techniques. *American Journal of Hospital Pharmacy* 1980;**37**:998-1005.

34. Peto R. Clinical trial methodology. *Biomedicine Special Issue* 1978;**28**:24-36

35. Peto R, Pike MC, Armitage P, Breslow NE, Cox DR, Howard SV, Mantel N, McPherson K, Peto J, Smith PG. Design and Analysis of randomized clinical trials requiring prolonged observation of each patient: I. introduction and design. *British Journal of Cancer* 1976;**34**:585-612.

36. Peto R, Pike MC, Armitage P, Breslow NE, Cox DR, Howard SV, Mantel N, McPherson K, Peto J, Smith, PG. Design and Analysis of randomized clinical trials requiring prolonged observation of each patient: II. analysis and examples. *British Journal of Cancer* 1976;**35**:1-39.

37. Schafer, A. The ethics of the randomized clinical trial. *New England Journal of Medicine* 1982;**307**:719-724.

38. Schoolman HM, Becktel JM, Best WR, Johnson AF. Statistics in medical research: principles verses practices. *Journal of Laboratory and Clinical Medicine* 1968;**71**:357-367.

39. Schor S, Karten I. Statistical evaluation of medical journal manuscripts. *Journal of American Medical Association* 1966;**195**:1123-1129.

40. Watson AB. Informed consent of special subjects. *Nursing Research* 1982;**31**:43-47.

41. Zelnio R.N. Data Collection Techniques: Mail Questionnaires. *American Journal of Hospital Pharmacy* 1980;**37**:1113-19.

The following additions are made to update the reading list:

BOOK:

Altman D: Practical statistics for medical research. Chapman & Hall 1991.

ARTICLES:

Bland JM, Altman DG. Statistical Notes:

    Correlation, regression, and repeated data. *BMJ* 1994;**308**:898

    Regression towards the mean. *BMJ* 1994;**308**:1499

    Diagnostic tests 1: sensitivity and specificity. *BMJ* 1994;**308**:1552

    Diagnostic tests 2: predictive values. *BMJ* 1994;**309**:102

    Diagnostic tests 3: receiver operating characteristic plots. *BMJ* 1994;**309**:188

    One and two sided tests of significance. *BMJ* 1994;**309**:248

    Some examples of regression towards the mean. *BMJ* 1994;**309**:780

    Quartiles, quintiles, centiles, and other quantiles. *BMJ* 1994;**309**:996

    Matching. *BMJ* 1994;**309**:1128

    Multiple significance tests: the Bonferroni method. *BMJ* 1995;**310**:170

    The normal distribution. *BMJ* 1995;**310**:298

    Calculating correlation coefficients with repeated observations: Part 1-correlation within subjects . *BMJ* 1995;**310**:446

    Calculating correlation coefficients with repeated observations: Part 2-correlation between subjects. *BMJ* 1995;**310**:633

    Absence of evidence is not evidence of absence. *BMJ* 1995;**311**:485

Brennan P, Silman A. Statistical measures for assessing observer variability in clinical measures. *BMJ* 1992;**304**:1491-4

Brennan P, Croft P. Interpreting the results of observational research: chance is not such a fine thing. *BMJ* 1994;**309**:727-30

Britten N. Qualitative interviews in medical research. *BMJ* 1995;**311**:251-3

Carpenter LM. Is the study worth doing? *Lancet* 1993;**342**:221-3

Campbell MJ, Julious SA, Altman DG. Estimating sample sizes for binary, ordered categorical, and continuous outcomes in two group comparisons. *BMJ* 1995;**311**:1145-8

Chalmers I. What do I want from health research and researchers when I am a patient? *BMJ* 1995;**310**:1315-8

Daly LE. Confidence intervals and sample sizes: don't throw out all your old sample size tables. *BMJ* 1991;**302**:333-6.

Datta M. You cannot exclude the explanation you have not considered. *Lancet* 1993;**342**:345-7

Editorial. Should we case-control? *Lancet* 1990;**335**:1127-8

Ernst E, Resch KL. Concept of true and perceived placebo effects. *BMJ* 1995;**311**:551-3

Fitzpatrick R. Surveys of patient satisfaction: I-Important general considerations. *BMJ* 1991;**302**:887-9

Fitzpatrick R. Surveys of patient satisfaction: II-Designing a questionnaire and conducting a survey. *BMJ* 1991;**302**:1129-32

Fitzpatrick R, Fletcher A, Gore S, Jones D, Spiegelhalter D, Cox D. Quality of life measures in health care. I: Applications and issues in assessment. *BMJ* 1992;**305**:1074-7

Fletcher A, Gore S, Jones D, Fitzpatrick R, Spiegelhalter D, Cox D. Quality of life measures in health care. II: Design, analysis, and interpretation. *BMJ* 1992;**305**:1145-8

Florey C. Sample size for beginners *BMJ* 1993;**306**:1181-4

Gore SM. The Lancet's statistical review process: areas for improvement by authors. *Lancet* 1992;**340**:100-2

Grisso JA. Making Comparisons. *Lancet* 1993;**342**:157-60

Glynn JR. A question of attribution. *Lancet* 1993;**342**:530-2

Johannessen T, Lewis JA. For Debate. Controlled trials in single subjects. *BMJ* 1991;**303**:173-4

Jolley D. The glitter of the *t* table. *Lancet* 1993;**342**:27-9.

Jones J, Hunter D. Consensus methods for medical and health services research. *BMJ* 1995;**311**:376-80

Keen J, Packwood T. Case study evaluation. *BMJ* 1995;**311**:444-6

Kitzinger J. Introducing focus groups. *BMJ* 1995;**311**:299-302

Korn EL, Baumrind S. Randomised clinical trials with clinician-preferred treatment. *Lancet* 1991;**337**:149-152

Leon DA. Failed or misleading adjustment for confounding. *Lancet* 1993;**342**:479-81

Mays N, Pope C. Rigour and qualitative research. *BMJ* 1995;**311**:109-12

Mays N, Pope C. Observational methods in health care settings. *BMJ* 1995;**311**:182-4

Mertens TE. Estimating effects of misclassification. *Lancet* 1993;**342**:418-21

Morton AP, Dobson AJ. Analysing ordered categorical data from two independent samples. *BMJ* 1990;**301**:971-3

Pocock SJ. When to stop a clinical trial. *BMJ* 1992;**305**:235-40

Pope C, Mays N. Reaching the parts the other methods cannot reach: an introduction to qualitative methods in health & health services research. *BMJ* 1995;**311**:42-5

Rothman KJ. Lessons from John Graunt. *Lancet* 1996; **347**:37-39

Rothwell PM. Can overall results of clinical trials be applied to all patients? *Lancet* 1995;**345**:1616-9

Silverman WA, Altman DG. Patients' preferences and randomised trials. *Lancet* 1996;**347**:171-4

Sitthi-amorn, Poshyachinda V. Bias. *Lancet* 1993;**342**:286-8

Stirrat GM, Farrow SC, Farndon J, Dwyer N. The challenge of evaluating surgical procedures. *Annals Royal Coll Surg Engl* 1992;**74**:80-4

Stone DH. Design a questionnaire. *BMJ* 1993;**307**:1264-6

Thompson SG, Pocock SJ. Can meta-analyses be trusted? Lancet 1991;**338**:1127-30

Victora CG. What's the denominator? *Lancet* 1993;**342**:97-9

Wager E, Tooley PJH, Emmanuel MB, Wood SF. Get patient's consent to enter clinical trials. BMJ 1995;**311**:734-7

Warlow C. Organise a multicentre trial. BMJ 1990;**300**:180-3

Wyatt JC. Acquisition and uses of clinical data for audit and research. *J of evaluation in Clinical Practice* 1;1:15-27

INDEX

The Author has been a medical statistician since 1979 and has worked with researchers from many disciplines in the design & analysis of medical research projects.